FOREWORD

The papers that follow were presented at the Third Invitational Conference of the National League for Nursing Committee on Long-Term Care and Ross Laboratories. Papers from the first and second conferences are published, respectively, in the volumes entitled *Creating a Career Choice for Nurses: Long-Term Care* (National League for Nursing, 1983) and *Overcoming the Bias of Ageism in Long-Term Care* (National League for Nursing, 1985).

Papers from the third conference are the results of discussions on State of the Art: Needs and Care of Older People, Increasing Nursing Awareness of Long-Term Care Options for Older People, and Initiatives in Addressing Health and Related Needs of the Elderly. This volume contains information on meeting the nutrition and housing needs of elderly persons, including educational programs, professional education, hospice programs, congregate living, and recent trends in management and funding of community-based programs.

Each chapter contains study questions and a reference list. The conference recommendations are also included.

ABOUT THE AUTHORS

Ethel Mitty, MS, RN, is director of nursing, Jewish Institute for Geriatric Care, New Hyde Park, New York.

Sister Anne Marie McNicholl, PhD, RN, RPT, is vice president for planning, Our Lady of Mercy Miseracordia Medical Center, New York.

Sylvia H. Schraff, MSN, RN, is executive director, Home Nursing Agency of Blair, Huntingdon, and Fulton Counties, Altoona, Pennsylvania.

Lou Anne Poppleton, MS, is director, Meridian Home Health Services, Baltimore, Maryland.

Michael A. Creedon, DSW, is the Andrews professor of gerontology, Center for the Study of Aging, University of Bridgeport, Bridgeport, Connecticut.

Sherry Kittelberger, MS, RN, is director, Medical Nutritional Nursing Services, Ross Laboratories, Columbus, Ohio.

Sister Rose Therese Bahr, PhD, RN, is professor, The Catholic University of America School of Nursing, Washington, D.C.

CONTENTS

Chapter 1   Institutional Long-Term Care:
                Nursing Role and Responsibilities   1
                Ethel Mitty

Chapter 2   Congregate Living and the
                Institutional Campus   9
                Sister Anne Marie McNicholl

Chapter 3   The Hospice Concept   15
                Sylvia H. Schraff

Chapter 4   Home Health Services:
                Organizational Dilemmas   23
                Lou Anne Poppleton

Chapter 5   Housing for Elderly Persons:
                Its Implications for Nursing   35
                Michael A. Creedon

Chapter 6   Health Care and Nutrition Services   45
                Sherry Kittelberger

Chapter 7   Professional and Public Education
                Initiatives Addressing Health and
                Related Needs of Elderly Persons   63
                Sister Rose Therese Bahr

                Recommendations   79

1 INSTITUTIONAL LONG-TERM CARE: NURSING ROLE AND RESPONSIBILITIES

Ethel Mitty, MS, RN

The traditional conception of long-term care, shared by both the public and the health professional, is that of an institution which "custodializes" the old people who cannot take care of themselves, or who cannot be cared for by others. This view is not changing because of an expanding social consciousness but because of a shrinking health care dollar. The continuum of long-term care is a marketing phenomenon which is affecting every sector of the health and wellness industry; it has also generated countless education programs.

Commonly, the need for long-term care is associated with the frail or "at-risk" elderly. However, it also includes a population under the age of 65 which ranges from preteens to the middle-aged; persons with a variety of chronic, disabling conditions secondary to disease or trauma. Since our focus is the geriatric client, I will limit my remarks to that segment of the populace.

Institutional long-term care is evolving into a two-tier system of intensity of care. Short-term stay is geriatric rehabilitation; long-term, or permanent care is the more familiar and prevalent nursing home. The acute care setting (i.e., the hospital) is discharging three types of elderly patient:

1. The patient requiring intensive, complex rehabilitation secondary to cerebral vasular event, large bone fracture, cardiac event, or major surgery.

2. The patient who requires semiskilled nursing care (alternate level of care); this is the patient who is terminal, or demented, or significantly physically or mentally compromised.

3. The patient who can be discharged directly from the hospital to the community, given adequate and appropriate formal and informal community supports.

It has been my observation that nurses do not know the difference between Medicare and Medicaid, third-party reimbursement, the uses and capture of private savings to pay for long-term care, the "Nursing Home Without Walls" program, or any of the other programs and regulations which affect the enabling and disabling consequences of bureaucracy on health care. As a result of this abysmal lack of information and knowledge, nurses' ability to manipulate the system and enlist the consumers' advocacy is severely limited. It is also obvious that the various nursing theories elaborated in nursing schools fall apart in the long-term care setting, primarily because of the type of record-keeping virtually forced on members of the nursing home industry by the state and federal surveillance protocols. Primary nursing is an underutilized function in the nursing home staffed with only 30 percent nurses, 10 to 20 percent of whom are licensed practical nurses. We are dooming the registered nurse to frustrated professional goals and ideals when we promulgate a primary nursing practice framework as the quintessence of the nursing art. We would do well to reconsider, as suggested by Zander (1985) and Stevens (1985), that primary nursing is the cognitive aspect of nursing: managing and planning, not necessarily "doing." (For the nurse who must supervise the care of 30 to 50 disabled elderly patients as provided by a staff of 70 percent nonprofessionals, primary nursing as currently practiced is a misnomer and a disservice to both the graduate nurse and the long-term care setting.)

THE RUGs PROSPECTIVE PAYMENT SYSTEM

The DRGs as a prospective payment system is matched by the long-term care prospective payment system known as RUGs: Resource Utilization Groups. For the nursing home or long-term care client, diagnosis is neither a good predictor of care needed nor of outcomes. RUGs groups patients into a case mix index based on activities of daily living, behavior, some medical conditions, and a few skilled nursing needs. Statistically deriving that the nursing resources used are a surrogate for all service use, RUGs consists of 16 patient groups arrayed within five hierarchies or patient typologies: *special care, rehabilitation, clinically complex, severe behavioral disorder,* and *reduced physical functioning.* Documentation in support of RUGs placement, case mix index, and the subsequent reimbursement requires that patient needs be described in terms of the actual resource used (i.e., care provided). For example, whether the behavior required a staff person to stop what he or she was doing to intervene; whether the event was predictable or unpredictable; and precisely how many times the behavior occurred in a four week period. The activities of daily living must be described in terms of the resource (i.e., staff) used 60 percent of the time, whether the nursing presence was assistive (i.e., hands on) or supervisory (i.e., "didn't touch"), and whether it was constant or intermittent. The paperwork screams which had abated for a short while (during which time we really concentrated on the caring process and outcomes and staff development) are now being heard loud and clear.

The long-term care RUGs prospective payment system proposes to offer incentives to the nursing home to admit the rehabilitation patient. Admitting this type of patient as soon as possible is a system payoff; it costs less to care for this patient in a nursing home than in a hospital. An additional incentive, assuming our prognostic accuracy, is to discharge this patient to a lighter level of care or back to the community, with or without formal supports, as soon as possible. Another incentive offered is to admit the heavy care or alternative level of care patient who will become a permanent nursing home patient and who always will be a heavy resource user. The rehabilitation patient needs skilled professional nursing care on a short term (8–12 weeks) intensive basis whereas the long-term care patient needs custodial care delivered by the non-professional; this patient, however, requires continuous professional nursing supervision and case management. The skill mix is rather broad. The situation is alarming when one looks at the small nursing home and some proprietary nursing homes which generally have only one registered nurse on each tour; the charge/medication nurse is an LPN. One of the ideas proposed by RUGs was that the dollars paid to the nursing home for "bed hold days" should be slightly reduced. This would discourage nursing homes from "dumping" patients in hospitals. I am concerned for the nursing director who is essentially told by the administrator or owner that patients are to be retained in the nursing home—regardless of the circumstances. The RUGs system has been in effect since January 1986. Early reports are that the voluntaries will have significantly reduced reimbursements; also, the incentive package has not been mentioned recently. The RUGs prospective payment system is being tested in several other states as a model for Medicare long-term care reimbursement. I would point out that the geriatric nurse practitioner is not recognized by the RUGs system, either as a provider or a "resource used."

New York State has a fairly rigorous quality assurance process to which certain RUGs criteria can be linked. If, in fact, nursing homes experience reduced reimbursement, or the frequency of rate adjustment does not keep pace with the case mix index, the capacity and willingness of a long-term care facility to admit and absorb certain types of hospital or community patients may be less human than what the system hoped for.

RELATIONSHIPS IN THE LONG-TERM CARE SETTING

The long-term care milieu is an extended family. The situations, events, and issues which confront any commune get acted out in the nursing home. The architecture, color and light, greens and glass which describe a home environment similarly apply to a nursing home. The intergenerational and cultural relationships that prevail in society are present in a nursing home. Lab and pathology reports are as important to family and staff interactions as birthdays, deaths, and holidays. Staff advocate for patient rights almost as vigorously as they do for their collective bargaining unit rights.

A piece of legislation which has had as much negative effect as positive is the Chapter 900, Patient Abuse, Mistreatment and Neglect Law. While it has compelled us to carefully scrutinize and vigorously follow up on all incidents and accidents (as a result of which, for example, transfer technique and use of physical restraints are better monitored) it has also set up an adversarial relationship between management and workers and between management and the regulatory agencies. In essence, this law charges you as guilty: the burden of proof, usually in the form of interviews and written statements from all staff, of not having been abusive, and so forth, falls on the care provider. The law also sanctions anonymous phone calls to report abuse, mistreatment, and neglect. A major thrust of staff development is the building of trust so that an event is reported to the nurse as soon as it occurs, without fear of discipline which might otherwise attend such a report. It is not uncommon for staff to refuse to work as a team because of fear of association with a marginal care-providing colleague. Furthermore, staff protect each other rather than openly discuss problems and issues in delivery of care. And while the Patient Bill of Rights is a most laudable protocol, staff have used it to avoid giving personal care, for example, by reasoning that the patient has a right to refuse to take a bath.

By far the most difficult area of professional practice is in the human relations between the professional and the non-professional (e.g. the aide, nursing assistant, orderly). Political, cultural, and economic variables are present in the clinical setting. Forms of skill upgrading such as teaching aides how to take blood pressures, shoe care and polishing, toileting care, gift-giving, all become issues of the job description, self-esteem, title, and salary. Nothing moves or changes in long-term care as quickly or as smoothly as management science or introductory psychology courses outlined or predicted. Because of the sparsity of colleagues, the nurse has few if any peers with whom to discuss nursing or patient care issues, or test out new approaches. A study of risk taking by nurses from different educational preparations was most interesting: the master's baccalaureate nurse was reported to be more of a risk taker than the diploma or associate degree prepared nurse (Gries & Schnitzler, 1979). Differences in leadership style and philosophy of care were observed between directors of nursing coming from different educational backgrounds. When we consider that most long-term care nurses are practical nurses, diploma, and associate degree graduates, and most directors of nursing are diploma grads who later acquired Bachelor's degrees (let alone a Master's degree), the implications for long-term care are profound. Therefore, the milieu to which we still actively recruit nurses may be quite different, from the theoretical as well as the experiential framework in which the nurse was educated.

The self-care movement is, of course, not new to long-term care. The commitment to personal dignity and autonomy went hand-in-hand with our concomitant fostering of dependency. In failing to recognize the residual strengths and restorative potential in our patients we have not been as alert to the depersonalizing and disengaging effects of institutional living. Territorial, acting-out behavior may be as much an expression of free-will as it is behavior reflecting fear and confusion secondary to a symptom of organic brain syndrome. The cultural expectations of the behavior of old persons also projects into the practice framework. Recent studies of elderly persons in the community find that self-reports of health status are related to activity level (McKracken-Knights, 1985). Despite the multiple chronic conditions and physical disorders associated with aging, subjects reported the ability to take care of themselves and be free from worry as healthy. Medical regimen compliance behaviors, particularly in relation to drug regimen compliance, show no clear relationship to the client's level of education or extent of knowledge (Sands & Holman, 1985). Compliance behavior is unpredictable by the usual variables and apparently diminishes as distance from the original learning increases. This is particularly important in regard to the rehabilitation patient whom we are discharging from the nursing home to the community. Our follow-up protocols are spotty at best; we have no data that identifies continuing compliance behavior. However, we do know two things. The elderly client both in the health care institution and in the community is subject to polypharmacy. Also, a significant number of the elderly require hospitalization because of accidental drug overdose. We know very little about socialization behavior in the elderly and what constitutes "normal" from "not normal" (Brown, 1968; Levine, 1969).

EDUCATION AND TRAINING NEEDS OF THE GERONTOLOGICAL STAFF

Rehabilitative nursing of the elderly client is not the same as that of other age groups. Prognosis measures are as different as the healing processes. A patient with below the knee amputation secondary to diabetes mellitus could walk again with a prosthesis, but only after cardiac status is stabilized and strengthened. While one would expect any person to be highly motivated to walk again, the older person will be terrified of falling. Attention span and ability to understand and follow directions are affected. The permutations of the care plan must also include the effects of dislocation trauma and the subclinical onset of depression. Clearly, the nursing plan of care is different; the intensity and kinds of resource use is different. Decubitus treatment is eclectic and represents, more and more so, shared research and resources of the hospital and the nursing home. With the entry of health maintenance organizations as Medicare-approved providers of care, the interest in short term intensive rehabilitation as a cost-effective locus of care will increase. Once the private insurance industry is assured of its profit margin, the approval already given to some insurance companies will be aggressively marketed.

The extended care facility and intermediate care facility are not and cannot be psychiatric facilities. Patients do poorly when they are removed from the psychiatric setting to a custodial or long-term care setting; facilities of this kind do not really have psychiatric support services. It is unrealistic to expect a long-term care facility staff to have that range and depth of skill and knowledge to be both a therapeutic psychiatric facility and a nursing home. Programmatically, they are different.

While the education and training needs of the RNs who will work in a gerontological setting are becoming more clearly identified and structured into the curriculum, the preparation of the gerontological aide is still neglected. Yet it is this staff who render at least two-thirds of the primary care and is in ongoing relationship with the patient and family. Therefore, the responsibility and burden falls to the unit nurse—not the inservice department (which is frequently staffed by only one half-time person, all that the code requires). Even though most long-term care facilities prefer not to hire new graduates (we need them seasoned, tempered and experienced in acute care first), the need for continuing education cannot be underestimated. There is no curriculum for gerontological nursing at the undergraduate or non-degree level which could possibly address the variety of issues of gerontological nursing and care of the elderly.

Physical assessment of the elderly client is not the same as it is for the younger person. No event is short-lived or of limited impact. For example, the ramifications of a single tooth extraction can be as follows: diet change, diminished food intake, signs and symptoms of infection, urinary tract infection secondary to decreased fluid intake, diabetic instability, and so forth. No less crucial is the knowledge and assessment skills for behavioral and cognitive indices. Language and communication must be modified for the client and the staff. Anticipating needs without infantilizing the patient becomes a fine art and a science.

The gerontological nurse of these closing decades is not the same as the nursing home nurse of even one decade ago. More than ever, the nurse is the team leader working with colleagues in other disciplines, particularly physical medicine and rehabilitation, social service, and medicine. Similar to a hospital setting, rehabilitation and admitting units work at a frenetic pace, and are well staffed with nurses who are equipped and trained to manage cardiorespiratory arrest. On the traditional long-term care unit, the tempo is slower; it is 60–80 percent staffed with aides, and many patients might be coded as DNR (do not resuscitate). The team approach to patient care plans and decisions includes all professional staff, aides, the patient if possible, and the family. In several facilities, the chaplain or pastoral counselor also participates in team meetings. Heretofore almost exclusively a hospital domain, committee participation (e.g., Joint Practice Committee, Nurse Practice Committee, Ethics, New Products, Safety and Risk Management, Infection Control, Pharmacy and Therapeutics), now occurs in the nursing home. It was an enlightening experience for me to ask my clinical staff whether they felt it was necessary to perform autopsy examination of the elderly patient. Most of them felt there was no need; "the patient died of old age."

Without question, marketing long-term care involves the gerontological nurse. Whereas formerly we were creative in ways to provide the best care, regardless of cost, we are now in an era of diminished resources and cost containment, struggling to meet our philosophical and professional goals within the context of productivity measures, quality assurance, and marketplace competition. The utilization of staff and supplies in today's highly regulated, fiscally constrained market requires a gerontological nurse who is both a case manager, people mover, and documentarian.

Research is desperately needed on measures of professional nursing effectiveness in long-term care (e.g., pain management, incontinence management, humanistic nursing, the quality of life, self-care effect, compliance behaviors). Nurses who will advocate for the elderly person from the perspective of long-term care services that must not be curtailed are needed. The role and function of the geriatric nurse does, in fact, vary with the setting and the type of client need. One perspective which is helpful is based on Barbara Stevens' (1984) proposed alternatives of independent nursing practice in relation to medicine. Her construct is (1) nursing has the same patients and the same goals as medicine; (2) nursing has the same patients but different goals from medicine; (3) nursing has different patients but the same goals as medicine; and (4) nursing has different patients and different goals from medicine. Given the nature of long-term care staffing (allotments imposed by the state), we are required to forge a functional assignment system with our holistic view of humankind. Nursing diagnosis is not completely adequate for care planning; it falls short on prognostication. If we abjure the medical model and medical diagnoses, we could endanger the patient's life. My point is that no one health discipline controls the patient and the outcomes; everything comes into play but the gerontological nurse is the conductor.

The challenge to long-term care participants is to reach out to the nurse, patient, and director of nursing services in the small long-term care facility. For every nursing home which closes, the discontinuity in long-term support for the aging population will be irreparable for generations. For every nurse who completes his or her education without the gerontological basics, and for every year in which NCLEX fails to include questions testing knowledge and skills of gerontological nursing, the profession abdicates its social contract with society.

REFERENCES

Brown, M.I. (1968). Social theory in geriatric nursing research. *Nursing Research, 17*(3).

Gries, E., & Schnitzler, B. (1979). Nurses propensity to risk. *Nursing Research, 28*(3).

Levine, R. L. (1969). Disengagement in the elderly: Its causes and effects. *Nursing Outlook.*

McKracken-Knights, A. (1985). Look beyond your client's answers. *Journal of Gerontological Nursing.*

Sands, D., & Holman, E. (1985). Does knowledge enhance patient compliance? *Journal of Gerontological Nursing, 11*(4).

Stevens, B. J. (1984). Nursing theory: analysis, application, evaluation. Boston/Toronto: Little, Brown and Co.

Zander, K. (1985). Second generation: primary nursing: A new agenda. *Journal of Nursing Administration, 15*(3).

STUDY QUESTIONS

1. We can describe the nursing role and practice in long-term care as scientific, technical, managerial, and interpersonal. Give an example of each role and describe how it may be different from nursing practice in the acute care setting, and in community home health care?

2. What patient outcomes can be expected and measured in the long-term care setting from the perspective of quality assurance? What are productivity measures in long-term care?

3. What is the special clinical knowledge that applies to gerontological nursing? What are the special skills?

4. Identify and discuss three clinical nursing problems in long-term care that need research. What are the criteria of informed consent for the elderly client?

5. Given the state of technology that is available in the long-term care setting, what are the issues involving ethics that come to bear? What is the nurse's role in making decisions on these issues involving ethics?

6. Discuss the interdisciplinary health team as a model for planning care in the long-term care setting. What are the education and training needs of the nurse assistant?

2 CONGREGATE LIVING AND THE INSTITUTIONAL CAMPUS

Sister Anne Marie McNicholl, PhD, RN, RPT

Congregate housing is a label applied to a variety of living arrangements for elderly persons. It is a life-style that has been in existence for approximately 20 years. Thus one generation of elderly persons have lived through this type of experience, and from them we have learned some very interesting facts.

Congregate living, depending on the geographic location or the sponsorship, could be anything from independent, age-segregated communities, apartment houses, and condominiums, to single-room-occupancy dwellings. They can offer basic services or full service.

According to published government reports from the U.S. Department of Housing and Urban Development, 95 percent of older Americans live in independent households and only five percent live in some type of institution. Because of the variety of definitions of congregate housing provided by the literature, it is difficult to say how many of these households can be classified as completely independent.

For the purpose of this paper I will use the operational definition of congregate living found in the government research, which reads: "Congregate housing is defined as age-segregated housing built specifically for the elderly (62 years and older) which provides, at the very least, an on-site meal program" (Ehrlich, Ehrlich, & Woehike, 1982). The meal program can be provided in a common dining room, a cafeteria, or the living unit. Various levels of congregate living are defined according to the functional levels required of the residents or the services provided to maintain independent living.

From all the information that can be obtained from the Department of Housing and Urban Development reports, we can assemble a profile of the congregate-living population. Primarily, they are white females. They have a significantly higher proportion of single and widowed persons than the national average and have a higher mean income than the elderly population at large.

9

They are more likely to have major health problems than the national elderly population. Congregate elderly see their housing as a place to grow old. Many have chosen congregate living because of health problems or social isolation. They are a group who have chosen not to live an entirely independent life-style; as they grow older they will seek an appropriate balance between their need for care and service and the attributes of conventional housing. Elderly persons who choose congregate living are looking for "care insurance." They want the security of knowing that care will be available and provided if and when they need it. The essential services they have identified are meals, nursing, medical, and housekeeping services.

There is an interesting disparity between the incomes of persons living in congregate housing and those of the national elderly population. Proportionately, those in congregate housing have incomes that are higher; however, the data also clearly show that their living expenses are higher. Social and recreational activities were given high priority in housing complexes with younger residents (ages 62 to 75).

TYPES OF CONGREGATE HOUSING

The following are the most common congregate-housing arrangements defined by the functional levels of their residents:

Independent.   Self-sufficient, able to shop, cook, and do household chores. Able to manage all personal care.

Semi-independent.   Requires some assistance with shopping, food preparation, and household chores. May or may not require assistance with personal hygiene. Could use the services of a homemaker.

Communal housing.   Varying range of services provided by contract for a monthly fee that is either included in the rental charge or separate. Usually includes household tasks and one or two meals per day. Usually has public recreation areas, dining room, and recreational activities.

Retirement hotel.   Similar to communal housing with the addition of hotel-like service and accommodations.

Personal care homes.   Provides personal care, housekeeping, meals, assistance with mobility, recreational programs and supervision. Residents are either physically, cognitively, or emotionally impaired.

Intermediate care.   Provides health care according to government definitions and standards.

Skilled care. Provides total care according to government definitions and standards.

Several or all of these facilities can coexist in an institutional campus. For most, the multilevel campus includes all levels of care ranging from minimal supervision to sophisticated levels of health care. Rarely is there a place for completely independent living in these complexes, and in many instances dependency is fostered. Where a continuum does exist, studies have found that the individuals who chose such an arrangement were usually planning ahead for the time that they would require more intensive care than they felt could be provided in their own home. They looked to this arrangement as a panacea.

There is a lot of uncertainty in the selection of the multilevel campus but that depends on the model chosen. Researchers have identified many of the shortcomings of congregate housing in their studies of two main models—constant and accommodating. The constant model remains the same and presumes that residents will remain totally independent. The accommodating model provides backup services and has plans for the individual's needs as they arise. To date, the data indicate that the turnover rate is higher and the tenure shorter in the constant model.

Most older people have at least one chronic condition (80% according to the National Center for Health Statistics, 1980) and for this age group multiple conditions are a common occurrence. As the nature and severity of these conditions affect older people's functional level, independence decreases and need for support services increases.

Of one thing we can be certain: "Whatever the initial level of health and coping ability that may exist in the original tenants of such housing, it can be predicted that over time the independence of some will decline. It can be further expected that elderly persons entering some years after the original tenants will will be characteristically different from the original group. Thus, as people change over time, the characteristics of their environment may also need to change" (Ehrlich, Ehrlich & Woehike, 1982). The likelihood of the need for institutional care can be kept to approximately 12 percent for this population if support services are available, accessible, and affordable.

RELOCATION

Given the current situation, the elderly persons living in housing on a multi-level campus have limited access to services in their homes and are moved to other levels of care on the same campus when the need arises. According to Rosswurm (1983) "Relocation is a potentially stressful event in anyone's life. For the older person, relocation is often preceded by declining health, financial problems, death of a spouse, and/or urban renewal. The changes in lifestyle that relocation brings can create stress in the older person whose homeostasis may be precarious." Because of the increase in stress that reloca-tion effects on an already unstable situation, "environments should be built for the adaption to the changing needs of older persons, rather than asking older persons to relocate as their dependency levels change" (Creedon, 1986). Ideally, this should be the model for the congregate living arrangements designed for the elderly rather than the norm of intra- and inter-institutional transfer that involves environmental change. Granted, intra-environmental change is less deleterious physically, emotionally, and socially; however, it does have a negative effect on the individual involved and requires the expen-diture of scarce energies to maintain his or her equilibrium. Although each level of care or each facility found on the multilevel campus ostensibly responds to specific needs, the specificity is more of an administrative convenience than a response to the specific needs of older persons.

A cost analysis of congregate living sites has shown that the sites where the fewest services were provided were those with the most positive financial status, and that those where the most services were provided were operating at deficits. Institutionally-based services are far more costly than services pur-chased from free standing providers because institutionally-based services reflect a more costly level of care with higher operating expenses and a larger debt service.

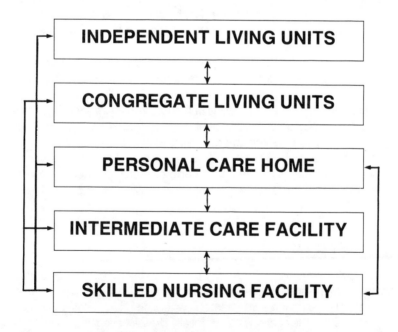

Figure 1. Schematic of the present situation.

THE ROLE OF THE CASE MANAGER

Ideally, the managers of congregate living units should contract or broker community-based services that would provide a holistic package. Managers should aim at educating the medical provider and the consumer about the appropriate and available linkages that maintain the older person's ability to remain in his or her own home. Support services include budgeting and financial planning, shopping, pet care, transportation, religious, homemaker–home health aide, nursing, health, social, counseling and recreation and socialization.

The role of the case manager is to facilitate the movement of clients from one service to another as the need arises, and to evaluate the effectiveness of the service. It is even possible to provide for the client with complex needs if there is a careful referral system and follow-up. A successful site also requires a communication system that ensures the transfer of necessary information to the providers of service. The key to its success is monitoring.

The case manager should be a professional capable of assessing the client's need and making judgments concerning the specific kinds of services that should be provided. In order to make the appropriate recommendations, the assessment must be comprehensive and provide reliable, accurate information. Improper or inadequate matching of services to the client's needs may result in a misunderstanding—older persons may feel the only answer to their problems is institutionalization.

High-risk screening is essential for identifying individuals requiring closer monitoring and more frequent evaluations. This will allow for preventive measures to be implemented and planning initiatives to be tested before there is a crisis situation.

For too long the needs of community-based elderly persons and those living in congregate housing have been neglected. Now there is a new awareness of a growing aged population that is expanding the health care market and creating the need for new services. There will be a highly competitive environment characterized by marketing strategies and profitability.

If health care professionals are to be identified as advocates of elderly persons and innovators of their care they will need to assume the role of case managers and develop the needed linkage with providers to form a regional network. If health care professionals do not take the initiative and establish standards and criteria for home care services that go beyond health care, we will be faced with an overcrowded marketplace positioned for profitability and continuing to leave essential gaps in the provision of service.

The expansion of the institutional campus to include congregate living arrangements is but one answer to the growing demand for alternative living arrangements for the elderly. To be viable and responsive to the growing population of "at-risk" elders sites need to be linked to a broad spectrum of services that are coordinated by a responsible manager. This would reduce the need for institutional care at all levels and would add a dimension of quality to our later years.

REFERENCES

Ehrlich, P., Ehrlich, I., & Woehike, P. (1982). *The Gerontologist, 22*(4), 386.
National Center for Health Statistics. (1980). *Monthly Vital Statistics Report.* (PHS)
     80–1120. U.S. Government Printing Office.
Rosswurm, M.A. (1983). Relocation of the elderly. *Journal of Gerontology, 9* (12),
     632.

STUDY QUESTIONS

1. What are some of the problems that force the elderly persons who live in suburban and rural areas to relocate?

2. What is desirable about congregate living? What is undesireable?

3. What is the ideal situation? How could our society move toward it?

4. What role can nursing play in keeping older persons in their own homes or in congregate dwellings?

5. What alternative living arrangements for the elderly exist in your area? Where are they located? What features would attract older persons?

3 THE HOSPICE CONCEPT
Sylvia H. Schraff, MSN, RN

Death is a part of the natural phenomenon of life. Healthy dying is as important a consideration as healthy living, yet most of the people in our health care system view death as a failure. Hospice is a concept that focuses on living while managing the physical, emotional, and spiritual aspects of dying. The hospice movement has helped turn our attention to the special needs of the dying and has given us the opportunity to bring comfort and support to those whose remaining life is limited.

The concept of hospice is not new; it is the revival of a humane, commonsense approach to an everyday occurrence. Hospice is a medieval term describing a place where travelers or pilgrims received shelter and comfort on their journey. Dr. Cecily Saunders is credited with the revival of the hospice as a place to provide care to the dying. Saint Christophers, in London, is a freestanding facility for the terminally ill. It was founded in the 1960s by Dr. Saunders out of the need to create an atmosphere where people could die with dignity and in relief of the pain associated with their illnesses. Likewise, Dr. Saunders is responsible for introducing the concept to the United States following her visit to the Yale–New Haven Hospital in Connecticut. Although based on the experience of Saint Christophers, the hospice movement in the United States centers around the home as the place of care in contrast to a specially designed facility. This unique twist on the movement resulted in myriad approaches when the hospice concept became popular during the 1970s.

Early hospice organizers were usually interested community people who were frustrated with the existing medical care system. Most of these early hospice programs were small and voluntary in nature, and emphasized the spiritual and emotional aspects of dying. Some of the programs operated within the health

This paper is dedicated to Edgar A. Stoltz, beloved husband of Nancy Stoltz, Assistant Administrator of the Home Nursing Agency of Blair, Huntingdon, Fulton, and Bedford Counties who died August 6, 1985 in his home after a lengthy illness. His efforts to live his remaining life to the fullest will continue to serve as an inspiration for staff, family, and friends for years to come. Ed exemplified the spirit and the philosophy of the hospice concept. He will always be in our memory.

care system, while others operated independently. As the television and print media began to cover the movement, interest started to grow especially among the health care providers. Professionals began to vie with the community volunteers for their right to be invovled. Workshops and literature were devoted to issues related to death and dying. Hospitals, nursing homes, and home health agencies developed separate programs and services to provide for the needs of the terminally ill. Soon it was apparent that if the movement was to survive, standards had to be developed, special interest groups needed to be unified, and a method of financing had to be developed.

In an attempt to bring some order to the progress being made, the National Hospice Organization was founded in 1978. Standards for hospice care were developed in a joint effort by the National Hospice Organization and the Joint Commission on Accreditation of Hospitals. The organization lobbyed Congress to provide funding for the care that was being provided. As a result of this pressure, the Health Care Financing Administration authorized funding of 26 demonstration programs in 1979 and the Tax Equity and Fiscal Responsibility Act of 1982 was amended to provide hospice benefits to Medicare eligibles. What had started out as an effort to bring about change in our methods of caring for the terminally ill evolved into a legitimate program of care recognized and funded by the government and private payer sources.

The National Hospice Organization's drive to enact hospice legislation was probably aided by the nation's growing interest in cost containment and by the changing attitudes about life and death. Rapidly rising health care costs spurred interest in alternatives to less costly institutionalization. Home care was an attractive cost-saving alternative. At the same time, people were asking for the opportunity to participate in decisions affecting their care. Home care, which involved family and community members, was perceived as a more humane approach to non-acute care. Hospice was indeed a timely movement which won the acceptance and support of many in a very short time.

As might be expected, a movement of this magnitude was not without its opponents. The movement began in response to the medical care system's inability to appropriately provide for the special needs of the dying. Lay persons, clergy, family counselors, and many others were frustrated in their attempts to ease suffering and allow death to occur in a familiar setting where the patient is surrounded by loved ones. Special interest groups developed outside the existing health care system. Within the system, there were those who were uncomfortable with any model of care that passively accepted death. Some argued that palliative care destroyed hope and created despair. Others felt that all resources available should be employed to prolong life for as long as possible. Moral and ethical dilemmas of both models of care were and will continue to be debated for years to come.

Today, hospice care has become an integral part of our health and human services system. There are approximately 1,500 hospices in existence. According to the National Hospice Organization, an estimated 100,000 people received the benefits of this new program during 1985. Within these programs, there are many variations. The General Accounting Office identifies five major models:

1. Freestanding hospice.

2. Hospital-affiliated, freestanding hospice.

3. Hospital-based hospice (a) acute-care hospital with centralized palliative care or hospice unit; (b) acute-care hospital hospice team who visit patients; (c) units operate as part of a Health Maintenance Organization.

4. Hospice within an extended-care facility or nursing home.

5. Home care program only (a) hospital-based; (b) nursing home-based; (c) community-based.

Variations exist within the models listed above. Some of the models depend solely on volunteer support and provide care in conjunction with existing resources. Others employ a case management model combining volunteer and paid staff who work with multiple organizations and providers to supplement care.

In order to look more closely at hospice, it is essential to understand some of the basic characteristics of the program. The National Hospice Organization defines a hospice as "a centrally administered program of palliative and supportive services which provides physical, social and spiritual care for dying persons and their families. Services are provided by a medically supervised interdisciplinary team of professionals and volunteers. Hospice services are available both in the home and in an inpatient setting. Home care is provided on a part-time, intermittent, regular schedule and around the clock on-call basis. Bereavement services are available to the family. Admission to a Hospice Program of care is on the basis of patient and family need."

Central to the hospice model is the provision of care that is described as palliative in nature. The dictionary defines palliate as "to lessen the severity of without curing; alleviate." Palliative care has come to mean care that focuses on comfort and support in contrast to care that is primarily directed at the treatment of the disease. It must be stressed that while comfort is the primary concern in this model of care, it does not preclude initiation of remedies to deal with the illness. The team's major goal is to ease the suffering that may be more than physical in nature, so that the dying person and his or her family will have the energy resources available to deal with future problems.

Rachel Spector (1984) stated that, "pain is the most critical symptom to control in the care of the terminally ill." She adds that "the pain is not only physical but also social, psychological, and spiritual." Hospice staff must be specially trained to ease the many pains of the dying and their families. Team members must be adept at helping people to express their feelings. Team members need to know how to help patients control physical pain and its disabling effects. They must be expert on the use and administration of available drugs and narcotics. They must help the patients and their families control the suffering so that together they have sufficient strength to plan for the future.

In addition to the concept of palliative care, hospice programs emphasize the special needs and functions of family and friends (the family is the unit of care). Central to this belief is that family members not only provide care to the patient but also receive support and comfort. Petrosino and Weitzel (1984) state that

> their involvement is important in meeting the needs of the patient; it also provides an opportunity for their own needs to be addressed. Thus, family members and friends become both providers and recipients of care.

Helping families face the inevitable, cope with the realities of the situation, and eventually pass through the grieving stage more constructively is one of the central concepts of hospice.

Another characteristic of hospice is the use of a team approach to the planning and delivery of care. This interdisciplinary team utilizes the talents and expertise of a number of professionals from a variety of backgrounds. Medicare regulations require the interdisciplinary team to be composed of at least a physician, a nurse, a social worker, and a pastoral or other type of counselor. Other team members that may be included are chaplains, nutritionists, physical therapists, occupational therapists, speech pathologists, home health aides, pharmacists, dentists, and volunteers involved in the care of the patient. Myra Downs (1984) describes the hospice team as "the clinical component of any hospice program." She also states that "the needs of a family facing the death of a loved one may be simple, requiring intervention by only a few members of the team, or complex, requiring at some time the work of all team members."

The use of volunteers is not new to the hospice movement, although it is rather unique to the health care system. From the initial stages of the movement, volunteers were considered an essential component to an effective program, not just an add-on. This basic concept of using volunteers to assist supportive staff and supplement the family as well as the professional caregivers has probably contributed more to the success of the movement than any other component. Pedersen (1984) points out that

> large numbers of well-trained volunteers, who augment the services of the professional staff are crucial to the existence of hospice programs, because hospice provides more than just good medical and nursing care.

Volunteers not only help within the program with their time and talents, but also assist in advertising the nature of the service. Often, community success is directly related to the image of the program described and promoted by the volunteers.

It is essential that hospice programs screens all applicants and provide train-ing for the potential volunteer. This early stage is important for both the volunteer and the program to ensure that unresolved emotional conflicts are recognized and that volunteers have the education to function effectively as members of the team. Most training programs are designed to last approx-imately four to six weeks. They cover aspects of death and dying, symptom control, communicating skills, use of community resources and bereavement. Participants have the opportunity to openly explore their own fears of dying as well as gain insight into their personal needs and future roles.

Bereavement services are another element of a hospice program. In the introduction to *Bereavement, Reaction, Consequence and Care,* Osterweis et al. (1984) state:

> the shapers of public policy and educators in the health professions also are becoming more concerned about bereavement's toll. There is strong and growing public interest in preventing stress related illness, including that which may be precipitated or exacerbated by grief.

The value of a well-planned bereavement service has been recognized since the beginnings of the hospice movement.

"The overall goal of any bereavement program is to help the individual or the family unit, to move toward resolution of their grief" (Demi, 1984). Hospice programs have adopted a variety of approaches to the provision of bereave-ment services. Some use only professional staff, while others offer a combina-tion of volunteers, community support, and professionals. As Demi (1984) points out, "What works well in one community may fail in another." However, because of the way the program is structured, it is essential that all persons involved know when to raise "the red flags that may signal a need for profes-sional mental health intervention and be knowledgeable about lay and pro-fessional community resources to which the bereaved can be referred as appropriate and desired" (Osterweis, et al., 1984).

One milestone in the evolution of the hospice movement was the enact-ment of the Tax Equity and Fiscal Responsibility Act of 1982 which amended the Medicare Program to include hospice care. According to the Department of Health and Human Services, "the goal of hospice is to help terminally ill individuals continue life with minimal disruption in normal activities while re-maining primarily in the home environment." The act helped to standardize hospice programs as well as provide a financial resource for them. Although the pros and cons of the legislation have been and will continue to be debated for years to come, the legislation was a recognition of palliative care as a legitimate model of choice for those facing impending death (Department of Health and Human Services).

A summary of the major provisions in the law follows. Parties are eligible if they are entitled to Part A of Medicare, receive prognosis of life expectancy of six months or less as certified by a physician, waive Medicare benefits for an elective period (two 90 day and one 30 day election periods are available), understand the palliative nature of hospice care.

An interdisciplinary group to supervise the care and services offered by the hospice program includes core services (nursing, medical, social, physician, counseling, and volunteer services and a quality assurance program) and other services (physical therapy, occupational therapy, and speech pathology; home health aide, homemaker, chore and companion services; medical supplies including drugs and biologicals; and short term inpatient care for symptom control and respite purposes).

The hospice reimbursement is limited to $6,500 per year aggregate cap per beneficiary. The following services are reimbursed:

Routine hour care. $53.17 for every day the client is at home under hospice care.

Continuous home care. $14.94 per hour for each hour of continuous home care provided after the first eight hours.

General inpatient care day. Maximum of $271.00 per day for acute or chronic symptom management limited to 20 percent of total days spent in the program.

Inpatient respite care day. $55.33 per day for caretaker relief (5 day limit).

Not all hospices in the United States elect to pursue certification under the new entitlement program. Many hospices rely on funding from philanthopic organizations, donations, memorials, grants and service fees, and are reluctant to change their programs to conform with the new regulations. However, innovative health care providers, seeing the potential in government funding, set up new hospices that satisfy the act's conditions for participation. The National Hospice Organization estimates that approximately 14 percent of all hospices have acquired certification as providers under the Medicare benefit.

I would like to share with you some of my experiences in developing a hospice program. The Home Nursing Agency is a large multicounty, voluntary, nonprofit, community health agency in south central Pennsylvania. The agency identified the need for a specialized care program for the terminally ill as a result of an analysis of the agency caseload and through discussions with staff, the Advisory Committees and related human services providers in the area. Following board approval early in 1979, the staff began by developing a philosophy of care, program goals, policies, and training courses. Staff attended workshops and continuing education sessions to ensure the program would evolve in accord with the national movement. Since the agency was already certified as a home health agency under the Medicare program, the hospice was envisioned to be an extension of that model. The agency had been utilizing specialized care teams for maternal and child services and felt a hospice home care team would be an appropriate and somewhat familiar approach for providing care to a select group of people.

As the program evolved, specialized policies and procedures were developed. The volunteer component was quickly recognized to be of utmost significance, and a training course was initiated at an early stage in the program's development. Bereavement counseling was originally provided by the professional nursing staff and later volunteers became adept at delivering this service.

Referrals came from a variety of sources including hospitals, physicians, health and human services agencies, clergy, family and friends. As the referrals increased, there was a corresponding increase in the staff's stress and anxiety from the affects of 24-hour availability of services; it became necessary to rethink the on-call system. It was decided that all nursing staff who took calls should receive a modified hospice training course designed to help them respond to the off-duty hour needs of dying. The effect of the effort was to greatly reduce the amount of stress and anxiety for hospice staff since the on-call rotation was reduced from once every three weeks to twice a year. Such a reduction in stress gave staff an opportunity to refine the program and gear up for the new hospice standards and certification.

In order to fully comply with the Tax Equity and Fiscal Responsbility Act (TEFRA) amendments related to certification, the agency found it necessary to add a hospice medical director and develop contracts with inpatient facilities for general and respite care. Contracts were also developed with pharmacies to supply drugs and biologicals at a prenegotiated rate. In turn, the pharmacies were required to deliver the medication and ensure 24-hour availability if necessary.

Today, the hospice program has evolved to include all four counties in our service area with contracts for inpatient care at local community hospitals and nursing homes as well as with local pharmacies. The entire multicounty program is coordinated through the hospice interdisciplinary team, which oversees the care provided and develops the policies and procedures for the program. Approximately 850 persons have been served through the hospice program since its inception only a few years ago. Community acceptance and patient satisfaction has far exceeded our original expectations.

At first, the financial aspect of the program was a detraction; its cost was high compared to the home health benefit. This was further compounded by the reluctance of the patients, staff, and physicians to elect the hospice benefits out of the fear of the unknown. As the program gained in experience, our staff's confidence grew in the new Medicare benefit. This resulted in more people electing to use the benefit. Today, the program is prospering both financially as well as in terms of its acceptance in the community. As we are confronted with a rapidly growing elderly population and a corresponding need to develop innovative approaches to provide for their needs, community-based systems of care seem to hold some promise especially in light of our country's thrust toward cost containment. Hospice is one community-based initiative that follows the current trend towards choice, responsibility for self, and max-imizing one's potential. "Death is not sensed as a defeat, but as a summation, a conclusion" (Reimer, 1974). It is through hospice that one can truly achieve this summation.

REFERENCES

Demi, A. S. (1984). Hospice bereavement program: Trends and issues. In S. Schraff (Ed.), *Hospice: The nursing perspective* (p. 135). New York: National League for Nursing.
Department of Health and Human Services, *Federal Register,* No. 56008.
Downs, M. J. (1984). The hospice team. In S. Schraff (Ed.), *Perspective* (p. 47). New York: National League for Nursing.
Osterweis, M. et al. (1984). Introduction. In *Bereavement, reactions, conse-quences, and care* (p. 4). Washington, DC: National Academy Press.
Pedersen, D. S. (1984). Volunteers. In S. Schraff (Ed.), *Hospice: The nursing perspective* (p. 18). New York: National League for Nursing.
Petrosino, B. M., and Weitzel, M. H. (1984). Role of the nurses. In S. Schraff (Ed.), *Hospice: The nursing perspective* (p. 95). New York: National League for Nursing.
Reimer, J. (1974). *Jewish reflections on death,* New York: Schocken Books.
Spector, R. E. (1984). What makes hospice unique? In S. Schraff (Ed.), *Hospice: The nursing perspective* (p. 7). New York: National League for Nursing.

STUDY QUESTIONS

1. Differentiate characteristics of palliative care from characteristics of the tradi-tional curative care model.

2. Describe the value of bereavement services in hospice programs.

3. Discuss the role of the volunteer in a hospice program.

4. Discuss the issues related to the hospice care movement.

5. Discuss the pros and cons of the Medicare hospice legislation.

4 HOME HEALTH SERVICES: ORGANIZATIONAL DILEMMAS

Lou Anne Poppleton, MS

We are in the midst of a nationwide organizational and financial health care revolution. This revolution will alter the patterns of medical care practice and consumer choices that we have known for the past forty years. As one commentator stated, "However the forces of change may be measured, it is clear that the movement of health care out of hospitals and into new places and forms will continue until what is left inside hospitals are the services that only hospitals can provide. The underlying reason it will happen is that this is what the people want" (Tresnowaski, 1985).

PROFILE OF AN AVERAGE HOME HEALTH AGENCY

The rhetoric of change should be grounded in the status quo. What does the home health agency of today look like? A recent survey done by the Subcommittee of Health and Long-Term Care of the House Select Committee on Aging identified a profile of the average home health agency today: its sources of revenue, its costs, services, and employees. The sub-committee found that the average agency:

- Employs 45 persons on a full or part time basis, equivalent to 27.5 full time staff.
- Employs an additional 6.7 equivalent persons to provide direct patient care by contract.

- Has eight volunteers who work 20 hours or less per week.
- Pays an RN an average salary of $17,493.
- Pays a home health aide/home maker an average salary of $8,886.
- Pays a director/administrator an average salary of $25,321.
- Had revenues of $486,875 in 1980 and $740,931 in 1982—a rise of 52 percent during that period.
- Has Medicare as its major source of revenue for 67 percent of its visits.
- Had a budget surplus in 1982 in 43 percent of the agencies; had a deficit in 41 percent of the agencies.
- Has budget costs of 65 percent in personnel areas.
- Provides 24-hour care in only about 66 percent of the agencies.
- Sees 1,407 clients, providing 9.6 visits at an average cost of $37.95 per visit, for an average entry cost of $364.32 per case.
- Has the largest group of clients in the 60–74 age category (35%).
- Has about 30 percent in the 75–84 age category with 11 percent in the 45–54 age category.
- Has a dominant ethnic background of white patients (64% are women).
- Treats the following most frequent conditions: diabetes, hypertension, heart/circulatory problems, cancer, stroke, arthritis, respiratory disease, and bowel, bladder and skin problems.
- Receives 48 percent of referrals from hospitals and 25.7 percent from private physicians.
- Makes 13,500 home visits.
- Records an average cost per client of $352.26 per month compared with $1,564 per month for the average nursing home, and $1,033 per month for custodial care (Health Care Financing Administration, 1985).

The per month costs may be an unfair comparison because nursing homes and custodial care also provide shelter, food, and recreational services as well as laundry in many cases.

THE RECENT GROWTH IN THE HOME HEALTH INDUSTRY

At least several factors have caused the growth and shifting patterns in the home health industry. These are:

- The unreimbursed, growing costs of institutional long-term care along with society's aversion to the nursing home environment.
- Consumer preferences for home care services.
- The entrance of women into the work force.

- The development of medical technology companies that have made the correct assumption that the applied medical technology explosion would lead to the need for "high-tech" patient equipment and skills long after the patient's acute-care phase.
- The need for hospitals to diversify their activities in order to capture and hold their market share of the community's at-risk population. Thus, corporate reorganizations, mergers, acquisitions, and joint ventures have become the pattern of growth and survival for today's medical and hospital care industries.

The following data quantify the impact of the above-mentioned factors on the home health industry. The number of agencies providing home health services has increased more than 20 percent each year since 1980. In December of 1984, the number of agencies in the United States totaled 5,300. By 1990, it is projected there will be about 8,000 for-profit agencies and hospital-based services—the two fastest growing types of home health agencies. Between December of 1983 and December of 1984 alone, there was a 57 percent increase in the number of Medicare-certified proprietaries and a 54 percent increase in the number of certified hospital-based agencies. A recent nationwide poll found that 70 percent of all hospital administrators either have developed or plan to develop a home care service. Administrators' attraction to these services is understandable. Through the home care service they are provided with a built-in source of referrals; they can gain financial rewards from offering additional services and equipment; and they can help to assure future readmissions from the home care contacts (Anderson & Louden, 1985). These are important functions for a hospital with a surplus of available beds.

As the numbers suggest, visiting nurse associations are being faced with severe competition. In some communities a hard-fought struggle for organizational survival is being waged. Government programs at both the local and state levels represent the minority of care givers—a significant shift from 1982 when they represented 50 percent of the total agencies.

Whether the shifts in organizational groupings will prove advantageous for patients and payers will be a question for future studies to explore. It does suggest to us now that, as in other areas of medical care, the patterns we have taken for granted for so long in home care services may not be viable. We must open our minds to new forms and functions if we anticipate being leaders in the planning and management of future in-home services.

Another way to visualize the impact of the recent growth of home care providers and services is to review the Health Care Financing Administration's (HCFAs) statistics regarding reimbursement of home health services. "Even though home health expenditures constitute only about 3 percent of overall Medicare costs, they are growing rapidly. From 1970 to 1980, Medicare reimbursements for home care increased at an annual rate of 34 percent. Since

1980, they have doubled from $772 million, to $1.5 billion in 1983, at an annual compounded rate of 26 percent. Increases in utilization accounted for the bulk of the reimbursement increase either through the increase in the proportion of beneficiaries using services, the increase in the numbers of visits per person served, or the growth in the number of beneficiaries'' (Health Care Financing Administration, 1985, p. 73). Medicaid experience with home health followed the same trend. For the five years ending in 1982, home health costs increased at an average annual rate of 23 percent (Interview with Margaret Heckler, 1983).

CURRENT DILEMMAS

So what are home health service providers complaining about? Isn't home health one of the few services predicted to undergo rapid change and continuing expansion for the foreseeable future? After all, groups such as Business Trend Analysts, Inc. project that the home health services and equipment market will increase to over $10 billion by 1995, making it one of the fastest growing segments in the health care industry (Business Trends Analysts, Inc.). Others see home health as an important way to reduce inpatient acute care patterns, thus resolving over-use and over-payment concerns that have become part of our national health policy debate. So what's the problem? Hasn't the home care industry yearned for this kind of support and recognition for years? The answer to this question is both yes and no.

It did not take much imagination to predict that HCFA would take an aggressive interest in the finances of this growing industry. That, in fact, is what happened and it leads me to some of the major problems that directly affect home care managers and home health services today.

1. *There is a strong adversarial stance between HCFA and the home health industry.* The elements of the argument are complex. Through Congressional testimony and other grievance measures the industry, which is represented in the aggregate by the National Association for Home Care (NAHC), the American Federation of Home Health Agencies (AFHHA), and the American Affiliation of Visiting Nurse Associations and Services (AAVNA/S), contends that the expansion of home care is systematically being curtailed at the very time when it could become the greatest cost alternative to institutional care. They (and others) charge that administration policies applaud and mandate deinstitutionalization, while they hinder home health agencies from providing services with budget cuts and restrictive reimbursement rules (Testimony to the House Select Committee on Aging, 1985). One measure seen as hindering home healthcare is HCFA's tightening of the regulatory definitions of "home-bound", "intermittent care", and "medical necessity." These definitions seem to be directed toward restricting access.

Additional actions include HCFA's recent reduction of available intermediaries, dropping the number from 47 to 10; its passage of restructuring regulatory cost limits that drop the Medicare caps for each of the next three years while instituting a "discreet costing" cap instead of letting agencies aggregate visit costs as they have done in the past; the instigation of a sharp increase in the denial of claims which reportedly comes in part from an HCFA contractural mandate with its intermediaries to produce at least a $5 return for every dollar expended in the medical review portion of the intermediaries' budget; the use of a sampling methodology for record review and visit denials which is then automatically spread across the agency as a whole (this has been reversed in at least one state through administrative proceedings); and HCFA's unsuccessful attempt to add a $4.80 co-payment for beneficiaries after the twentieth visit.

All of these recent HCFA promoted activities (as well as others not mentioned), are seen as ways to discourage the growth of home health services and to reduce the current numbers of home care providers. The concurrent questions must be—are these measures necessary to help police or clean up the industry or are they intended to use home health (never more than 3% of the Medicare budget) as one vehicle to decrease overall Medicare spending? Are they really intended to limit access to the elderly who need additional skilled help in the home in order to achieve their rehabilitative potential? Or are the restrictions necessary to help legislatures at both national and state levels differentiate between legitimate medical and rehabilitative care needs that are legal within the legislative requirements of Medicare and the social/personal care needs that are not part of the 1965 Medicare legislation. HCFA representatives suggest that the latter is true.

2. *The generic, nondifferentiated use of the term "home health" and its identification as a "hot ticket" item may work against the development of logical, definitive, reimbursable, systematic, nomenclature of noninstitutional acute and long-term care services.* As a nation, we easily grow impatient with policy "quick fixes" that don't work. My concern is that too much attention has been focused on home health as an economic panacea for more costly institutional care. Because the family, or the provider has had, up to this point, few reimbursement options other than Medicare to help shoulder the economic burden of medical or rehabilitation needs, the service definitions that Medicare uses have been stretched. It is not uncommon within my own agency to teach staff how to describe or document a situation in order to maximize the potential for reimbursement. If this situation is not ameliorated by appropriate reimbursement to support systems, study after study will continue to report that home care is not more cost effective than institutional care. Indeed, some situations cannot be more cost effective. The criteria for these situations should be differentiated, documented, and used for guidelines. Only when reimbursed personal care services, coupled with appropriate and reimbursable medical care services are recognized and accepted as a reasonable approach to the ongoing needs of individuals and families outside of institutional care, will individuals have appropriate home care options available to them. Without this enlightened policy approach, institutions in financial distress will increasingly be willing and able to document that home care doesn't work and that reorganized and renamed institutional care does work.

3. *Practitioners who offer guidance regarding the need for post-discharge institutionalization must be restricted so that the patient is not placed into an institutional setting long before he or she needs to be there.* Elaine Brody (cited in Cantor, 1985) writes that most older people need no more help than is given to them by family members on a day to day basis. She states that the young old, 65–74 years (60% of the aged population) are relatively fit and have little needs for intervention by anyone except in times of crises.

The next moderately old group, 75–84 years (30% of the aged population) have increasing rates of illness and disability, yet one-half have no limits in carrying out the activities of daily living. The oldest elderly, ages 85 and over (9% of the aged population) are the most vulnerable and need the most assistance (e.g., extensive personal care, shopping, supervision of medical regimes).

Taking these three age levels into account, the majority of experts believe that one-third of the elderly (about eight million people) need some help (Cantor, 1985). After a serious illness or trauma, the individual is at the highest risk of being entered into a nursing home. Primarily, this happens because of poor, last minute discharge planning, often triggered by the physician on the same day the patient is to be discharged. This last minute approach is inappropriate and shallow. Well-meaning caretakers and family members often cannot gather their resources for home care that quickly, so the patient may go to a nursing home or other institutional environment. Without aggressive advocacy, appropriate planning, and proper rehabilitation services the patient may not be able to leave the institutional care setting once admitted.

The long-standing pervasive myth that the elderly are isolated and abandoned without meaningful kin relationships has been destroyed by study after study. What has emerged is an extended caretaker system promoted by family, friends, and other kinds of caretakers, supported to some extent by formal organizations. Since we know that last minute discharge planning doesn't meet the needs of the patient or the family why do we continue to do it? If we acknowledge that some people need help and time to convert former self-sufficiency into semi-dependence, why does discharge planning with the family or caretaker not begin for high risk groups at admission to the acute care setting?

4. *It is my contention that as the physician's income drops, he or she will bring all but the most homebound individual back to his or her office for medical treatment.* The danger is that this narrower perspective of need will minimize the other services such as rehabilitation or personal care that the patient might also need. In the past, services have been thoughtfully combined in a carefully written medical care plan (usually initiated by the home care nurse), which the physician reviewed and signed. This plan allows continuity of care among and between a range of necessary multi-disciplinary practitioners and services. As was recently stated in Home Health Line, "Physicians as well as hospitals are seeing revenue decline as a result of DRG's. Many are moving into the home care market—because they are losing dollars in their practice." One administrator points out that, "Our average length of stay dropped one day (after DRG's), that's 40,000 MD visits or 120,000 consultant visits. At $50/hour that would in the aggregate, over a period of time, decrease physicians incomes by $6 million . . . They are scrambling for that patient post-hospital dollar" (Home Health Line, 1985, p. 79).

5. *The home care industry brings problems upon itself by insisting that the present and future mirror the past.* The field of home care, still a dependent service, must change with the times. Mergers, joint ventures, altered service groupings, high-technology nursing and other variations to an older, more structured, historical theme must be pursued and implemented whenever possible. If home health is to remain viable as an integral concept of coordinated aftercare services, members of the industry need to comprehend the options for change in the context of the changes occuring in all phases of medical and institutional care services. The industry must shrink itself to a core, that which cannot be changed or altered without giving up quality and responsiveness to in-home patients' needs. On the other hand, it must expand itself to do business in a changing forum to encompass other needs such as pediatric home care, health maintenance organization (HMO) and preferred provider organization (PPO) contracts, ventilator dependent services, and possibly care of the victims of acquired immune deficiency syndrome (AIDS), as well as other local or regional needs and opportunities.

Fortunately, there is Congressional hope and help for home health patients. On May 21, 1985, Senator Orrin Hatch (R-UT), Senator Edward Kennedy (D-MA), Senator John Heinz (R-PA), Senator Paula Hawkins (R-FL), Senator Bill Bradley (D-NJ), and Senator Robert Stafford (R-VT) introduced S.1181 the

Home and Community Based Services for the Elderly Act of 1985.
The bill would establish a block grant to provide funds for states to:

1. Coordinate all community and home health services currently pro-
    vided through a myriad of local, state, and national government
    programs.

2. Identify ways of assisting elderly individuals or groups at risk of in-
    stitutionalization in order for them to stay at home and in their
    communities.

3. Educate public, medical, and social work professionals about the
    services available to the elderly.

4. Encourage involvement of families, and voluntary, religious, and
    community organizations.

5. Provide basic home and community services to keep those at risk
    of institutional care in their homes.

6. Provide information to the Secretary of Health and Human Services
    for use in developing an analysis of cost effective methods for pro-
    viding home and community services.

Senator Kennedy in his statement accompanying this bill stated:

Home and community-based health services are not only humane, they
are cost-effective. Minimal and relatively inexpensive support services
can often prevent costly and debilitating episodes of illness and
hospitalization. Even higher intensity health services can often be
rendered less expensively in the home than in institutions. It is both wrong
and wasteful to require people to enter nursing homes to get the health
care they need simply because alternatives are unavailable or because
financing arrangements make non-institutional solutions infeasible.

In her statement, Senator Hawkins discussed the health care crisis in the
United States:

One of the few bright spots in this picture is the growing utilization of
home health care services. Not only is this a much more humane method
of providing care to the elderly, it is also far more cost-effective than
hospitalization or institutionalization. Home health care organizations,

whether they are affiliated with hospitals, hospices, nursing homes or free standing entities, have proved that they can provide quality cost effective health care.

Despite the obvious benefits of home health care, we have faced a difficult struggle in Congress convincing the Office of Management and Budget that extension of Medicare coverage to home health care services will reduce overall health care costs in the long term.

This short-sightedness has prevented passage of similar home health care legislation in the 97th and 98th Congress. With the implementation of DRG's causing a discharge of sicker and sicker patients, coupled with the increased aging of our over 65 population, the situation is even more acute. These patients need and deserve increased access to this humane and cost-effective form of health care. We as a nation facing a budget short-fall cannot afford to not enact this legislation. We must take action now to improve the access to home health care for our nation's elderly.

On June 11, 1985, Senator Bill Bradley joined by Senators John Glenn (D-OH) and Lawton Chiles (D-FL) introduced the Medicaid Home and Community-Based Services Improvement Act, S. 1277.

This bill is also designed to give the States more flexibility in providing home care services to persons at high risk of institutionalization. The proposal would terminate the waiver approval process for Medicaid Section 2176 waivers and would allow States, at their option, to provide home care services to Medicaid-eligible elderly and disabled persons to avoid institutionalization.

The bill also would increase by $150 a month the amount that a person can receive through family income before having to pay for home care services.

In his remarks introducing this legislation, Bradley stated:

We have to come to grips with the fact that long-term care is going to cost this nation a lot of money as the population ages. I believe that more home care—as an alternative to nursing home care services—is a humane and cost-effective approach. This bill allows states much greater flexibility to test out ways to provide affordable long-term care services at home.

Hawaii recently approved a law that allows payment for personal care services up to 65 percent of the average monthly Medicaid payment for a recipient in an intermediate care facility (excerpts from the National Association of Home Care's newsletter, 1985).

Two other influences may help to clarify the differentiation of services and the need for broader reimbursement models:

- The 18-million-member American Association of Retired Persons (AARP) will announce the specifics of a private insurance plan covering chronic or debilitating conditions as part of a huge group health insurance program for members. Working with Prudential, plans are being developed for reimbursed, in-home personal care and skilled services. The care will have to be ordered by a physician as a necessity for keeping an individual out of a long-term care institutional setting (Home Health Line, 1985, p. 137).

- Health insurance companies and employers are looking at reimbursed home health services as an alternative to hospitalization. A new era of benefit plan management seems to be evolving, which rewards patients (employees) who minimize the use (cost) of hospital care by accepting shorter hospital stays and in-home and support services.

There are 25 health insurance companies offering long-term care policies to the elderly. An article in the December 24, 1984, issue of *Business Insurance of New York* urged several groups to aggressively substitute home care for hospital care. They will soon publish hard data and anecdotal experiences to confirm greater savings through home care than institutional care (Thomas, 1985).

These possibilities for public-minded (e.g., AARP) and business interests to help stabilize the reimbursement base for selected groups of people brings hope to the problems that agencies and patients will face during HCFA's restrictive and cost-cutting phases.

The field of home care is changing in equal proportion to the overall changes in the health and human service systems. Much is expected of it, while the reimbursements support and historical professional support from individuals and institutions are not only decreasing but are becoming increasingly competitive in the market place. Home care programs are going to need to be creative while they aggressively pursue new relationships and new programs which will help guarantee their survival.

REFERENCES

Anderson, John A. & Louden, Teri L. (1985, January). Aging mix changing. *Home Care.* pp. 79–80.

Business Trends Analysts, Inc. Market Brochure (undated).

Cantor, Marjorie H. (1985). Families: A basic source of long-term care for the elderly. *Aging.* U.S. Dept. of Health and Human Services, Administration on Aging. No. 349. (Brody is quoted extensively in the article.)

Exerpts from the National Association of Home Care's Newsletter to members. (Fall, 1985).

Health Care Financing Administration. (1985). *Health Care Financing Review.* 6 (3), 73.

Health Care Financing Administration. (1985, May). *Home Health Journal.*

Home Health Line. (1985, March 25). *10,* 79.

Home Health Line. (1985, May 13). *10,* 137.

[Interview with Margaret Heckler, HHS Secretary]. (1983, November). *Home Health Journal.*

Testimony to the House Select Committee on Aging. (1985, August). *Home Health Journal,* pp. 1–3.

Thomas, Daniel. (1985). Trends in third party reimbursement for home care. *Caring.* 4 (6), 42–43.

Tresnowaski, Bernard R. (1985, February 27). *The Wall Street Journal.*

STUDY QUESTIONS

1. How have the recent changes in the health care system influenced the organization and delivery of home health services?

2. What impact does the generic use of home health terminology have on the industry? On patient care services? On legislation?

3. How can the efficient use of home health services lower hospital costs?

4. How does "professional over-help" influence long-term care practices? Do you think the concept is real?

5. Describe an "ideal" referral system for appropriately used home health and other long-term care services.

5 HOUSING FOR ELDERLY PERSONS: ITS IMPLICATIONS FOR NURSING

Michael A. Creedon, DSW

M. Powell Lawton summarizes 20 years of involvement in housing for the elderly with the statement,

> The good news is that over 20 years, we've seen two million older persons become housed in special housing that promoted their independence and enriched their lives. The bad news is that in the future, that number will grow primarily among those who can pay.

A new crisis in housing for elderly persons is developing rapidly. The growing number of persons over 75 years of age is increasing the absolute numbers of dependent elders while the federal government effectively ceases to support the development of section 8 and section 202 housing for the elderly. Current federal policy espouses a "voucher" approach to the housing needs of the poor and the frail elderly. Obviously, such an approach has its advantages, but one may question the ability of many frail older persons to effectively utilize the marketplace. In the absence of a public sector commitment to the shelter of frail elderly persons, the private sector faces a tremendous challenge in the immediate future.

Local housing authorities and zoning boards could begin to respond to this crisis by insisting that all future town development be predicated on 'mixed use' concepts. Shopping centers, department stores, office buildings could all incorporate some housing for older persons. While this may not be an ideal solution for everyone, one advantage is that elders would be close to the major transit lines and stores, another advantage is the spreading of the costs of housing elderly people. The present tax advantages of investment in office buildings and similar projects could be augmented with local tax concessions. Careful planning could also site such mixed-use facilities so that older people could have easy access to drug stores, food stores, doctors' offices, and similar service locations of particular relevance to elderly individuals.

While we address the need for specialized housing for the elderly we must think particularly of their long-term needs. Much has been written concerning the ill effects of relocation on older persons. Mirotznik and Ruskin (1985) discuss inter-institutional relocation and observe that relocations that involve moderate environmental change tend to have little negative effect on psychosocial status, while those involving radical environmental change tend to be deleterious to that status. The major point I wish to make here is that environments should be designed to meet the changing needs of older persons, rather than asking older persons to relocate as their dependency levels change. Thus, new housing for the elderly should include ramps, corridor and bathroom rails, and spaces that could be adapted as nurses' stations when and if necessary. I feel it is essential that nurses become strong advocates for adaptable environments. Nurses are and will be the frontline health care professionals as we move toward a community rather than hospital-based health policy. Associations must involve their members at the grass roots level in the process of shaping appropriate living environments for old people.

HOMEOWNERS

While many old people will not be able to live independently, the great majority of elders own their own homes. Currently some 75 percent of elderly people who head households in the U.S. are homeowners; it is expected that the homeowner population will reach 80 percent by the year 1995 (Pitkin and Masnick, 1981). Many of these homes are headed by females, most of whom are widows. Indeed, Newman (1985) estimates that by 1995 almost half of the elderly people who head households will be female. That fact becomes more ominous when we realize that some 49 percent of older women do not drive.

One of the most worrisome realities of today is the graying of suburbia. Large numbers of persons are retiring in the suburban houses they bought in their child-rearing years. For instance, Fairfax County, Virginia, has seen more than 100 percent growth in its over-65 population during the last census period. Inhabitants of the suburbs are notorious for their dependance on the automobile. Housing tracts frequently are located miles from shopping, health care, schools, and other amenities. The demographic data cited above give clear evidence to the projection that transportation will be a central problem for older persons in the years ahead. Local transportation systems must adapt to this need; hospitals, churches, and other major social institutions must develop supplemental transportation systems of their own.

The visiting nurse association is one nurse-sponsored health organization that has been at the vanguard of home care. We must vastly expand our home care services and recognize that older people will seek to remain in their own homes as long as possible. In this time of great transition in the health care industry we have unique opportunities to influence the health care system. Some hospitals are establishing geriatric outreach programs, others are contracting with or buying home care agencies. This is a favorable moment to encourage nursing professionals to become entrepreneurs and develop their own home care services. While nonprofit groups such as the VNA are doing great work, we must admit that the profit motive can produce a greater quantity of services more rapidly than any other method. The New York Times (1985, July 21) reported that the Drug, Hospital and Health Care Workers Local 1199 (AFL-CIO) in New York City has organized some 19,000 home health care workers and intends to retrain hospital workers for administering home care.

What does home care imply for the nursing profession? An enhanced appreciation of the psychological and social meaning of the home in the lives of elders should be a result of the new emphasis on home care. In the past we have too blithely focused on institutional health care as the core health care location, perhaps because of our faith in medical technology. Today we may be entering a new era where keeping people in their own environment is the appropriate alternative, not hospitalization. Most elderly persons own their homes, and the majority of older homeowners have lived in these homes for more than 20 years (Howell, 1985). These locations have an importance for their residents and are a reflection of their lives. In fact, Millard and Smith (1981) reported that the amount of time physicians and nurses spent speaking with nursing home patients directly correlated with the amount of personal memorabilia at the patients' bedside. We may therefore hope that home care will be enriched by a greater awareness of the unique history of the individual and a greater appreciation of their ways of coping.

Nursing schools could foster such awareness by requiring courses or at least modules on ecological factors in health care. We are all familiar with the medicine cabinet stories in which nurses, social workers, and other home care providers find large quantities of medications stored up, often outdated, frequently prescribed by diverse physicians, sometimes from different pharmacies. We need to be aware of the impact that lighting, seating, (a frail person in a house where there are no chairs with armrests, for instance), floor covering and bathroom facilities can have on the health of home care patients. Nurses must be able to assess these and many other salient features of a home as they visit the elderly person.

Perhaps just as important as a proper assessment of the environment is knowledge of the availability of resources for the environment's enhancement and the reimbursability of those resources. For example, there is a new armchair that shifts position electrically to enable an older arthritic person to rise to a standing position easily. The advertisement for the armchair is accompanied by an assurance that this piece of furniture is reimbursable through Medicare. Publications such as the *Journal of Gerontological Nursing* should frequently review such devices and report on their utility and (no less important to a fixed-income population) their eligibility for reimbursement.

Apart from coursework which would emphasize home care assessment, we need to refocus nursing education so that nursing students see elderly clients in their home settings. At the University of Bridgeport, nursing students have an opportunity to visit and provide care to elders in their homes. Professor Marsha Goodwin, of the Catholic University of America, organized a very successful volunteer health screening project at two apartment buildings in Washington where elderly people reside. Under her supervision, nursing students provided preventative health care to residents. It may be that all schools of nursing are now providing such opportunities to students. It certainly seems that all schools should make such programs a mandatory feature of the curriculum.

Reverse mortgages are a new and very important resource for the older homeowner. More than 70 percent of elderly persons own their homes and for the majority of them the home is their primary asset. There is now a wide range of banks, savings and loans, and other financial institutions that can arrange reverse mortgages. The reverse mortgage is based on the assessed value of the home and provides the owner with an income over a designated period of years while the bank obtains ownership of the home over that period. Obviously, this use of their major asset requires a solid grasp of the financial implications and many older people will need a good deal of counseling from trusted professionals. The nurse who visits elderly people in their homes, or who arranges health services for them, is often the person with whom old people share their worries about health costs.

Older people will sometimes refuse health care because they fear that the cost of the service or the medications will be exorbitant. Reverse mortgages can be an important solution for such fears. Therefore, there is an urgent need for nursing professionals who work with elderly persons to familiarize themselves with requirements for a reverse mortgage in their own state and make cash-poor persons aware of this important source of income. As we move toward the year 2000 the proportion of elderly persons who own their homes will approach 80 percent. While Medicaid and Supplemental Security Income eligibility rules do not consider the home as a source of income, elderly people and in particular those who refuse welfare assistance can alleviate financial distress and pay for health services through creative use of this major asset.

RELOCATION

The late Monsignor Geno Baroni was an Assistant Secretary of the U.S. Department of Housing and Urban Development during the Carter administration. Baroni had many years of experience in dealing with the housing needs of the poor and elderly people. He emphasized the needs of the 60-year old sons and daughters of elderly persons. These offspring must often care for college children and frail parents simultaneously. As health care professionals, nurses must educate the "children" of elderly persons about their own health care needs. Quite often such offspring are more anxious and guilt-ridden than the elderly parent. Adult "children" may press for premature institutionalization or they may pressure parents to abandon their lifelong home in order to move in with them. Such pressures, even with the best of motives, can frequently be destructive of both the autonomy and the physical and mental well-being of frail persons (Creedon, 1984).

On the other hand, frail elderly persons may sometimes need objective outsiders and health care experts to persuade them that they need care they cannot obtain at home. In either event a sound assessment of the person–environment fit is essential. One corollary is the need for communication skills for coping with families in crisis. We know that 83 percent never discuss with their elderly parents what to do in the event of a health crisis. Perhaps the most important contribution we can make is to protect the autonomy of the older person and ensure that he or she is the central decision maker at such a time. As numerous writers about relocation have stressed, when older people have choices about where they will live, when they have a chance to meet personnel from nursing homes or congregate living sites before their placement, then transition is much easier on them (Mirotznik & Ruskin, 1985).

The nurse can do much to ensure these opportunities are provided. Carol Schreter (1984) discusses home sharing as one of the ways in which old people can adapt to the loss of spouse, income, or health. This option seems to have great potential for the future when we consider the likelihood that many older women will be living alone in relatively large homes. A major obstacle to successful home sharing is the fear among older homeowners that they could not control their environment after accepting a home sharer. A network of honest brokers is needed for the future. Churches, civic organizations, perhaps even the VNA could offer matching services. Old homeowners could be matched with a houseseeker, with the understanding that the arrangement would be reviewed after three or six months, and new arrangements could be ensured for both parties. It seems clear that many elderly persons are reluctant to share homes because the fear that they will have to remain in a situation that they may dislike. Patrick Hare (1985), a nationally known expert on accessory apartments, suggests that the bulk of marketing by real estate agents, the rehabilitation industry, and the savings and loan associations, is also a major obstacle to homesharing. Perhaps nurses may not be the best placed professionals to broker such housing options, but they certainly can suggest or promote homesharing as a way to preserve the viability of an old person remaining in the community. Nurses can also alert homesharing groups to likely candidates for help.

While still on the subject of elderly persons who own homes, it is important to note the extensive literature on family and other informal support systems for the community-based elder. Shirley O'Bryant (1985) suggests that neighbors be included among such support systems. The nurse who provides community care should be familiar with this literature. Persistent efforts to locate children, relatives, and sympathetic neighbors may be necessary. Older people have specific preferences regarding who shall assist them. Cantor (1979) proposes a hierarchical composition model for this preference structure, while Dono et al. (1979) propose a task-specific model in which the nature of the task determines who might be asked to help. Sensitivity to the preferences of the older person combined with assiduity in the search for informal support systems are essential for the effective professional.

RURAL ELDERLY PERSONS

The rural elderly also generally own their own homes. The catastrophe in the U.S. farm belt over the past two years has been a particular misfortune for elderly individuals. First, the dramatic decline in the value of farmland has diminished the life savings of many. Second, the disastrous farm economy has accelerated the drift of younger generations from the farms. Hence, the rural elderly are much poorer today both in financial and in social support systems.

Rural elderly persons frequently delay in seeking health care until their condition becomes urgent. Consequently, they are often sicker than urban elderly persons when they arrive at the hospital. Likewise, rural elderly persons are more isolated, especially those who live on farms. The present drive to reduce hospital stays and to reward hospitals through the Diagnosis Related Groups (DRGs) prepayment system puts a great deal of pressure on the hospital staff to release old people early. It is essential that the existence and quality of community support systems be incorporated in discharge plans and that such factors be incorporated in reimbursement formulas. Dean Rosemary Donley of Catholic University and nursing leaders in Connecticut noted in a recent symposium at the University of Bridgeport that nursing factors are not reflected in the DRG reimbursement rates. It seems clear that the amount of support in the home environment must also be considered. An old person released from the hospital to a home where he or she has children and perhaps grandchildren available to help, is in much less jeopardy than one who returns to a home with a frail spouse and no other immediate supports. Quadagno (1978) notes that 17 percent of elderly people live in rural nonfarm settings while 5 percent live on farms. While most homes of rural elderly people have electricity, one in three lacks basic plumbing, a similar number lack a telephone, and some even lack central heating (Carp, 1976). Quadagno (1978) states that the rural poor are the most impoverished segment of the older population; they live in the poorest housing and they are the most isolated.

One of the ways we can respond to the health care needs of rural old people is through modern technology. Vanderslice (1985) describes a successful program in rural Texas where electronic monitors and phone units allow elders to live alone in their own homes. This project is funded with Title III funds under the Older Americans Act and the Texas Department of Human Resources. The project links local health providers—the informal support network (family, neighbor or friend) and other community providers such as members of the police, fire, and sheriffs' departments.

We need to foster such multidisciplinary and formal–informal support system links in all settings, not just rural communities. Some time ago I led a case-management training program in Washington, D.C., where social workers, nurses, and others in the case management system met with police and fire department personnel. Rarely does cross-disciplinary health care include these central community care providers. Nurses must be trained about these community resources and their specific roles and powers. For instance, a frail elderly person with Alzheimer's disease might not admit a nurse or social worker into his or her home, while refuse and unsanitary conditions make her a danger to the community. In such cases the nurse must be able to call on the appropriately sanctioned provider who can effect a forced entry if necessary.

We must insist that community support systems be a part of health care for rural elderly persons and we must develop methods to measure the capacity of the family and other informal support systems to provide home care. These measures must become part of our DRGs reimbursement system. If this does not occur we are in great danger of repeating the tragedy of the community care movement in mental health which has resulted in much deinstitutionalization and precious little community care.

This paper has not considered the health care needs of upper income elders. Such persons can and will purchase services as needed. One may only suggest that nurses enter the entrepreneurial home care field and offer a gamut of services to these people. We must build up evaluation systems if such entrepreneurial activity increases. It is not enough that the care providers be nurses. This very vulnerable population must be protected from fraud or abuse. The use of professional bodies that monitor the practice of their membership must be implemented.

Likewise, the paper has not considered the unique problem of minority groups. As Anne Towne, director of hospice for Washington, D.C., commented in recent correspondence with me, Oriental families may place a great taboo around the use of a home (or room) where an old person has died. Such cultural taboos obviously affect the health care system for older people, and on our efforts to maintain them in their own homes. Such an example reminds us that cultural, ethnic, and religious sensibilities of major ethnic groups must be addressed in geriatric nursing education.

Members of the nursing profession have a central and pivotal role in shaping the health care system. In their effort to lend it appropriate contours, active lobbying at all political levels as well as effective monitoring of what is currently provided is necessary. Finally, members of the nursing profession must be responsible for the development of models of care which can be cost-beneficial while accurately reflecting the support systems and needs of frail old people.

REFERENCES

Carp, F. M. (1976). Housing and living environments of older people. In R. H. Binstock & E. Shanas (Eds.), *Handbook of Aging and the Social Sciences.* New York: Van Nostrand Reinhold.

Creedon, M. A. (1984). Parish community involvement in meeting housing needs: An interview with Geno Baroni. *Social Thought, 10*(1), 51–59.

Hare, P. H. (1985). Accessory apartments: Who can afford to market the concept? *Generations, 9*(3), 43–45.

Howell, S. C. (1985). Home: A source of meaning in elders' lives. *Generations, 9*(3), 58–60.

Millard, P. H. & Smith, C. S. (1985). Personal belongings: A positive effect. *The Gerontologist, 21,* 85–90.

Mirotznik, J. & Ruskin, A. (1985). Inter-institutional relocation and its effects on psycho-social status. *The Gerontologist, 25*(3), 265–270.

Newman, S. G. (1985). The shape of things to come. *Generations, 9*(3), 14–17.

O'Bryant, S. L. (1985). Neighbors' support of older widows who live alone in their own homes. *The Gerontologist, 25*(3), 305–310.

Pitnick, J. & Masnick, G. (1981). *Projections of housing consumption in the U.S., 1980 to 2000, by a cohort method.* U.S. Department of Housing and Urban Development.

Quadrango, J. (1978). The impact of communal thought and values upon societal notions of aging and the aging's notions of themselves. pp. 48–55. In L. Foerster (Ed.), *The Aging in Rural Mid-America: A Symposium.* Lindsborg, Kansas: Bethany College Publications.

Schreter, C. (1984). Residents of shared housing. *Social Thought, 10*(1), 30–38.

STUDY QUESTIONS

1. Discuss the role of physical environment in the maintenance of independent living.

2. When would congregate living be an appropriate choice for the older person?

3. Reverse mortgages can be a useful tool to keep elderly persons at home. Discuss some of the problems you might face in helping an older homeowner get such a mortgage.

4. What aspects of the home are most likely to need upgrading for the physically disabled elderly person?

5. Discuss the nursing home as an appropriate setting for the frail older person.

6 HEALTH CARE AND NUTRITION SERVICES

Sherry Kittelberger, MS, RN

This paper discusses issues and initiatives related to meeting the nutritonal needs of the elderly in the community. An overview of older adults' nutritional status and needs is presented, followed by examples of initiatives which address these needs. The focus is on the presentation of the issues and discussion of priorities with recommendations for future planning.

OLDER ADULTS' NUTRITIONAL STATUS AND NEEDS

Several surveys have attempted to identify the nutritional status of the elderly as a group. The Health and Nutrition Examination Survey (HANES) (U.S. Department of Health, Education, and Welfare, 1977) and the Ten State Nutrition Survey, 1968-1970, (U.S. Department of Health, Education, and Welfare, 1972) surveyed the diets of older adults and identified deficiences in calcium, vitamin A, iron, vitamin C, and calorie intake. NHANES II (1976-1980) (Fulwood, Johnson, Bryner, et al., 1982) also identified declining nutrient intakes with age. Calcium intake was low for both men and women; iron intake was low for women. Calorie intake differed with income level and living arrangement; it tended to be higher in the rich and in those who lived with someone else. Protein intake was adequate. Another study (Betts & Vivian, 1985) rated the dietary adequacy of 100 noninstitutionalized older adults. Only one-third of the diets were rated as adequate. The nutrients most likely to be inadequate were calcium and vitamin A, similar to the results of the other surveys. These two nutrients were also the most likely ones to be inadequate even in individuals who were using vitamin and mineral supplements. One-third of the supplemented diets were deficient in at least one nutrient.

Some factors that are thought to influence the nutritional status of older adults include psychosocial status, educational level attained, mobility, special diets, cultural and religious affiliations, chronic illness, medications, and income. Individuals who are lonely or depressed are less likely to take in adequate nutrients. Immobile individuals have more difficulty obtaining and preparing food. Those with special diets, chronic illness, or numerous medications may have any number of problems related to decreased appetite, food intake, or absorption. Additionally, making appropriate, nutritious food choices within a limited budget is certainly possible but may be a formidable challenge to individuals with limited knowledge of nutrition.

The physical effects of aging also influence the nutritional status of older adults. Many older adults experience decreased biting and chewing ability because of lack of teeth or ill-fitting dentures. Decreased saliva production as well as a decreased sense of taste and smell may contribute to decreased appetite. Changes in the esophagus and hiatus hernias are other frequent occurences in the older adult population. Digestion and absorption may be influenced by changes in the older person's gastrointestinal tract.

Betts and Vivian (1985) looked at the effects of functional capacity, social and economic resources, physical and mental status, prescription medication use, ability to perform activities of daily living, and knowledge on nutrition status of older adults. Although each variable was statistically significant, these variables accounted for only a small portion of the variance in dietary adequacy. There are probably other variables which have yet to be identified. Futher study is necessary to determine how much influence these known factors have on nutrition, and what other variables are involved.

The usual standards used for nutrient needs are the Recommended Dietary Allowances (RDAs). These are defined as

> the levels of intake of essential nutrients considered, in the judgment of the Committee on Dietary Allowances of the Food and Nutrition Board on the basis of available scientific knowledge, to be adequate to meet the known nutritional needs of practically all healthy persons (National Academy of Sciences, 1980).

COMMUNITY NUTRITION PROGRAMS—PRESENT STATUS

The congregate meal sites and home-delivered meals are the major nutrition programs that meet the needs of older adults in the community. However, before discussing those options, there are other programs and special needs which should be pointed out. Most communities have sources of emergency food supplies at community action centers, church food pantries, and other voluntary organizations. Homemaker services for older adults may be obtained through community nursing services or the Department of Welfare. These homemakers assist with shopping and food preparation. Daycare services for older adults residing with relatives who work assure nutritional care through the day. For older adults with financial difficulties, food stamps may be helpful. Educational materials related to nutrition can be obtained through a variety of sources, such as the County Extension Service, Dairy Council, American Diabetes Association, American Heart Association, and State Department of Agriculture (Hentzler & Henneman, 1980).

Another special need for some individuals is for tube enteral or total parenteral nutrition (TEN or TPN) in the home setting. The number of patients receiving enteral nutrition in the home is increasing, and reimbursement is an unresolved issue. At present, one of the requirements of third-party payers is documentation that the "home enteral nutrition is a life-sustaining therapy rather than a food supplement" (Bennett, 1984). The Health Care Financing Administration (HCFA) is now in the process of developing guidelines for appropriate administration and cost. One problem for some patients is that they can eat some food normally, but they need a tube feeding to meet the majority of their nutritional needs. These tube feedings are generally not reimbursed because they are considered supplementary. Guidelines for TPN are also being developed by HCFA since increasing numbers of patients who cannot be fed enterally are going home on TPN. Wateska, Sattler, & Steigler (1980) examined the statistics of Cleveland Clinic patients on TPN, looking at costs of home and hospital care. They found that the average maintenance cost for the home parenteral patient was $54 per day, while the average maintenance cost for TPN in the hospital was $202 per day, a 73 percent difference. Statistics like these may be helpful in working with third-party payers.

Coordination of services is essential for patients going home on either TEN or TPN. Careful patient selection and teaching is needed before hospital discharge, and follow-up care is needed in the home. Folk & Courtney (1982) list the major issues which need to be considered in planning home care tube-feeding programs. These include setting criteria for selection of patients, obtaining the cooperation of a local tube feeding equipment retailer, establishing a patient–family teaching program, finding ways of obtaining third-party reimbursement, and continuing patient monitoring following discharge. Since most patients are hospitalized before progressing to a home nutrition program, it is often the hospital nutrition support service that initially coordinates these services and care and may also coordinate the follow-up. However, in many situations, once the patient is discharged, he or she is working with a community nursing service, a home health agency, and a durable medical equipment dealer.

The major community programs that respond to the nutritional needs of older adults include the congregate meal sites funded primarily by Title III-C of the Older Americans Act and home meal delivery funded in a variety of ways, including Title III-C of the Older Americans Act, Title XX of the Social Security Act, and private funding. Following several demonstration projects, the Nutrition Program for Older Americans began in 1972 when Congress authorized funding to meet the nutritional and social needs of individuals age 60 and older who could not obtain an adequate diet due to low income, limited mobility, or isolation. This was funded under Title VII of the Older Americans Act and provided for nutritionally adequate meals (one-third the RDAs) in senior centers, churches, or other appropriate settings. Services included outreach, transportation, health care, information and referral, health and welfare counseling, nutrition, and consumer education. The program has continued, and in 1978 it was combined with other programs under Title III to make it part of the Comprehensive and Coordinated Services Delivery System (Greene, 1981). The most recent revisions to the act were added in 1984. Title III of the Older Americans Act provides for a wide variety of services for older adults. The purpose is to develop and implement comprehensive and coordinated service systems, including supportive services, nutrition services, and multipurpose senior centers. Title III-C relates specifically to the nutrition services (U.S. Department of Health and Human Services, 1984).

These nutrition programs are geared to serve individuals age 60 and over and their spouses. There is a particular emphasis on low income of elderly persons. Additionally, there is an emphasis on promoting socialization, not just nutrition. Each component is important. The nutrition part of the program requires a hot meal or other appropriate meal at least five days per week containing one-third of the current RDAs for vitamins, minerals, and calories. To promote socialization, many sites carry out a variety of creative activities such as special theme parties, birthday parties, picnics, entertainment, games, dances, and service projects. Nutrition education and health promotion activities are also part of the program. These are implemented differently in different communities. Regardless of what form the programs take, older adults should be involved in planning. A registered dietician should also be involved with the nutrition education component and a registered nurse should be involved in the health promotion activities, although this is not mandated. The 1984 revisions of the Older Americans Act provide for demonstration projects related to education. These are discussed in the education portions of this paper.

Comments from program participants attest to the value of these centers. For example, a variety of persons involved in centers in the Akron, Ohio, area share some of their experiences (Mobile Meals, Inc., 1983):

- "We have in our center an 83-year-old amputee who is also a diabetic. If it were not for the Dining Center meals here, she would probably have had to have other living arrangements. Because the median age of the residents is 84 +, the meals have made it possible for many persons to maintain their independence."

- "I had surgery and lost 12 pounds. Your cheerful, friendly center has brought good nutrition for renewed strength and a fresh start on life."

- "A couple moved into the apartments on Friday. On Sunday, he was taken to the hospital and then to a nursing home. She became worn out going to visit him and was admitted to the nursing home. Eventually she became strong enough to go home, and the doctor said he would release her if she would eat in the Dining Center daily. She does; she gained 5 pounds in 3 weeks. Her personality has become much brighter; she takes seconds, smiles, and laughs. She volunteers, and last week stayed for a sing-a-long."

- "The good nutrition is an important concrete benefit to the participants, but the companionship and interaction between the seniors is also very important. For many of the participants, the Dining Center offers the only daily contact with other people, the only outlet for expressing their worries, joys, or sorrows of that day."

Another beneficial aspect of these programs is the use of older adult volunteers. Centers use older adult volunteers in a variety of ways. For example, Mobile Meals of Akron provides opportunities for older adults to serve as assistant food handlers, receptionists, outreach workers, members of the clean-up and menu planning committees; assist with presenting educational programs, escorting those without transportation, delivering home meals, planning publicity, representing Mobile Meals at public meetings, health fairs, and exhibits, and many other activities. The older adult volunteers are a valuable part of the program and they demonstrate that this is truly their program. The feeling of usefulness and self-esteem resulting from these volunteer activities is documented in a quote from one of the Akron Centers: "Mrs. C. is a widow and a very regular volunteer at our center. Volunteering gives her that special place to feel needed and useful. It gives meaning to an otherwise lonely life."

ISSUES RELATING TO COMMUNITY NUTRITION PROGRAMS

Five major issues related to existing community nutrition programs will be discussed here. These include funding of services, safety and sanitation issues, nutrient standards, nutrition education and health promotion, and outreach. Dietitians and nutritionists have been and should continue to be greatly involved in the resolution of many of these issues. Nursing should become more involved in two ways: supporting dietitians in obtaining the regulations needed to provide the best possible nutrition programs for older adults in the community, and in assuming a leadership role in the resolution of nursing issues relating to all of these concerns.

Need for Services and Funding Alternatives

In this age of prospective payment and DRGs (diagnosis related groups), earlier discharge of hospital patients into the community is already being seen and is likely to become more evident. Community programs need to be equipped for more comprehensive services and a greater number of clients. Coordination of these services is essential. The American Dietetic Association (ADA) (1984) identified funding and administration as priority issues in a position paper developed for Congress in 1984. One of their strong recommendations was that nutrition services be targeted to individuals who are at nutritional risk. Income level must not be the only criterion for nutrition service eligibility. As noted earlier, there are certain other factors which cause an individual to be at nutritional risk (e.g., living alone, decreased mobility, minority status, frailness).

Whenever possible, it is desirable to serve these high-risk individuals within a congregate meal setting in order to promote socialization and decrease social isolation. Thus, it is important to identify the areas in the community where older adults are most likely to congregate. Senior citizen centers and churches are rather obvious choices. A less obvious choice is put forth by Barbara Helwig (personal communication, July 1, 1985), director of Mobile Meals of Akron. She suggests that a breakfast site could be established at a local shopping center where a large number of senior citizens spend time each morning walking for exercise. Outreach to high-risk older adults and provision of transportation are important components of the program; funding must provide for these activities. Community health nurses could have a large role in identifying individuals in need of these nutritional programs and in encouraging them to attend. Obviously, the nurse should be aware of the programs in his or her area and also the potential areas where congregate sites need to be established. Nursing must lobby for adequate funding for these programs. There is little documentation of whether or not nutrition makes a difference in cost of health care. Together, nurses and dietitians should gather to provide that documentation.

Another controversial area related to the funding of these programs is the senior's contribution for the meal. Congregate sites provide a means for individuals to make a private contribution. There is some discussion about whether or not a specific amount should be requested in order to increase contributions, and how these specific contributions can be requested without discouraging individuals who cannot afford to pay. There is a danger of causing the very individuals who are at the highest nutritional risk to avoid congregate meals because of an inability to meet the requested contribution.

While funding of congregate meal sites has provided five nutritional meals per week for many mobile older adults, homebound individuals are not served as adequately. The problem is insufficient funding to provide services for all individuals in need. Many home delivery programs have long waiting lists; it is likely that people are eating very little while awaiting service. Hearings by Senator Ted Kennedy (1983) provided testimony that "the need for [congregate home-delivered] meals was double or triple the number that could be served at present funding levels." As individuals are being released from hospitals earlier, the need for home-delivered meals increases. Patients are going home sicker and less able to care for themselves without adequate community support. Increased funding for these programs is needed. Third-party payers generally do not fund nutrition unless the individual is completely dependent upon tube enteral nutrition or total parenteral nutrition.

Obviously, methods must be identified to meet the needs of the homebound individual who cannot cook for herself or himself and has no one else who can do so on a regular basis. This need applies not only to older adults but also to younger homebound patients. One recommendation from ADA (1984) is that transfer of funds from congregate to home-delivered meals be encouraged. There is some provision for this in the Older Americans Act.

Creative programs may be another means of obtaining needed services. For example, one hospital in Columbus, Ohio, has a contract with the Community Health and Nursing Services Meals on Wheels program to provide home-delivered meals to patients in need of this service and discharged from that hospital. The hospital will pay Meals on Wheels for the meals and then bill the patient. This is meant primarily for a short-term patient. This cooperative program enables the Meals on Wheels program to cover the costs involved. Thus, more individuals are served. Another pilot program that is federally funded and includes home-delivered meals is called Passport. This program is aim at individuals below a certain income level who would ordinarily go to a nursing home but with adequate community support can remain in their own home (M. P. Howley, personal communication, July 8, 1985).

There is also a need to carefully assess individuals' needs for home-delivered meals, and this is certainly an area where the community health nurse may be involved. Individuals who are candidates for congregate meals sites should not be receiving home-delivered meals, not only because of cost but also because the home-delivered meal does not provide the opportunity for socialization, education, and other activities associated with the congregate sites. The need for home-delivered meals should be assessed in terms of individuals' ability to meet their nutritional needs over the weekend. Some individuals need to have meals delivered seven days per week. Most will do well with delivery of meals five days per week, leaving the weekend the responsibility of a son or daughter, other relative, or friend. By gaining the assistance of someone close to the patient, the homebound patient is not isolated from loved ones. In fact, if meals are delivered seven days per week, other contacts with friends and relatives may tend to be less frequent, resulting in further isolation. Obviously, each family situation needs to be assessed individually.

However, some families and friends may not be willing or able to assist, in which case meals may need to be delivered seven days per week. Care must be taken that the homebound patient does not spend weekends without eating. Program funding must be sufficient to provide for these individuals.

Safety and Sanitation Issues

Safety and sanitation of food for both the congregate sites and the home-delivered meals is a concern. ADA identified their position on this in 1984:

> Specify minimum standards for food temperatures and holding times, and compliance with federal, state, and local health and safety laws and regulations, in the Act. This is essential to prevent foodborne illness, which could seriously threaten the lives of participants.

Obviously, this is also a concern of nursing. At present, there are no federal regulations regarding food safety and sanitation for either the congregate sites or the home-delivered meals. State or local regulations are supposed to cover these programs, but in many areas, no one is watching. Areas that have central kitchens and knowledgeable staff have more control over food handling. However, in areas where food is cooked and handled in numerous small, local kitchens (e.g., churches and schools), there is less control. Careful training of staff and volunteers is essential so that food holding and the transportation of food can be accomplished safely. Federal guidelines may improve standards.

Nutrient Standards

RDAs are not always an accurate tool for the assessment of the nutritional status of older persons. It should be kept in mind that RDAs are averages for populations, and specific requirements for an individual may differ from the RDAs. The older adult population in particular presents a problem because there is insufficient data about their nutrient needs. The adult RDAs for vitamins and minerals are divided into age groups 23–50; 51 and over. However, this does not take into consideration the changes that most likely occur in nutrient needs as individuals age and body composition and processes change. The nutrient needs of a 60-year-old may be quite different from those of an 85-year-old. Unfortunately, data do not exist to answer the question of what these differences are. We do know that energy needs decrease with aging as the resting metabolic rate and physical activity decreases. Thus, adult RDAs for calories are divided into those males and females in age groups 23–50, 51–75, and 76 and over.

The National Academy of Sciences is in the process of updating RDAs and has called for some changes, including a lowering of RDAs for vitamins A, C, B_6, magnesium, iron, and zinc and an increase in RDA for calcium. They are also proposing a change in definition of RDAs to "the levels of essential nutrients needed 'to protect practically all healthy persons against nutritional deficiencies' " (National Academy of Sciences, 1980). There is some controversy over these proposals. One area of controversy is that the definition change seems to lead to a narrower concept of RDA, one that is less focused on health. Additionally, if the RDAs are decreased, then there could be fewer nutrients required for federal nutrition programs, such as Meals on Wheels and school lunch programs (Pear, 1985). At present, these RDA revisions are on hold.

In addition to the problems with standards for nutrient needs, there are similar problems with identifying standards for nutritional assessment. The effects of aging on height and weight, body proportions, and distribution of body fat makes it difficult to interpret nutritional assessment data. Additionally, it is often difficult to obtain accurate measurements in nonambulatory individuals. Chumlea, et al. (1985) identified a methodology for obtaining accurate body measurements in older adults regardless of mobility status. This study also provides reference data to be used in evaluating nutritional status and intervention.

Further issues for discussion include:

- Fewer calories are needed as aging occurs and lean body mass, basal metabolism, and activity all decrease (Hickler & Wayne, 1984).

- Protein needs are in question since amount and distribution of body protein changes with age (Munro & Young, 1978).

- Calcium absorption and metabolism and its relationship to osteoporosis is a continuing area for controversy and study; there may be a need to raise the RDA for postmenopausal women and elderly men from the present 800 mg per day to as high as 1,500 mg per day (Freedman & Ahronheim, 1985; Albanese, 1978).

These are only a few of the questions still to be answered for older adults. ADA's (1984) recommendation is that the present standard of one-third the RDAs be maintained as the minimum per meal requirement for the congregate and home-delivered meals programs; that menu planning and meal supervision by a dietitian/nutritionist be required; and that project sites serve meals at least five days per week with one project site per area providing for home-delivered meals seven days per week.

Nutrition Education and Health Promotion

In addition to nutrition services, the Older Americans Act provides for supportive services that include nutrition education and health promotion activities. ADA's position is primarily related to nutrition education and recommends that it be mandated and funded as a separate line item; that qualified dietitian/nutritionists plan, develop, and evaluate nutrition education experiences; and that program participants be involved in planning nutrition education activities (The American Dietetic Association, 1984). Indeed, in the 1984 revisions of the act, a separate provision was made for health and nutrition education. The act provides for at least one demonstration project for health and nutrition education in each state after September 30, 1986. Each project is to be administered by the area agency on aging, in consultation with a gerontology center and may be in conjunction with a school of public health or medicine or voluntary organization. The programs are to be designed to improve the health and nutrition of older adults through physical fitness activities and nutritional improvement (U.S. Department of Health and Human Services, 1984, p. 27). Gerontological nursing departments of colleges or schools of nursing may want to consider working with other health professionals on these demonstration projects since the health and nutrition education would best be a multidiscipinary endeavor.

Aside from the future demonstration projects, nurses should be involved with health promotion activities. These activities may include such things as health screening and assessment, information on health risks (e.g., hypertension and stress), and the need for physical activity. Many congregate sites arrange to have nurse speakers for these various roles and topics. Nurses in the community need to become actively involved in these programs. The problem is lack of funding to reimburse nurses for these services. Additionally, documentation is needed to demonstrate that nutrition education and health promotion make a difference in the health of older adults. Nurses should take an active role in such research.

Outreach

Since the nutrition programs are established to serve high-risk older adults, it is necessary to find ways to reach these individuals and encourage attendance at congregate meal sites. Outreach workers are employed by many nutrition sites. Schneider (1979) identified barriers to effective outreach. One barrier was fear on the part of older adults. They feared adventuring outside of their accustomed living pattern. They were often reluctant to answer the door when approached by an outreach worker who was a stranger. Some of the outreach workers expressed fear for their own safety in entering dangerous neighborhoods; they tended to avoid those areas. Obviously, community health nurses already in these neighborhoods can play a large role in working with older adult clients to encourage attendance at congregate sites. However, improved organization and implementation of existing outreach programs is needed. Environmental factors were also identified by Schneider as potential barriers. Some individuals would not attend sites identified with a particular racial group, while others were reluctant to attend sites in churches of a particular denomination. Additionally, if the programs were perceived as "welfare," some older adults avoided attendance. Other individuals were so isolated that no one knew about them (e.g., those living in hotel rooms or sleeping on park benches). Inadequate transportation to sites was a problem. Location may also be a barrier if sites are not located strategically near the most needy older adults. Schneider made several recommendations to overcome these barriers:

- Targeted neighborhoods should be thoroughly surveyed before a nutrition site is established so that there is a basis for establishing the site.

- Outreach workers should be organized in pairs and should reflect the race, sex, and age balance of the area.

- A decision to use a church as a site should be given careful consideration. Churches can be excellent resources for finding program participants, even if they are not used as actual sites.

- Cooperative agreements should be developed so that outreach efforts could use existing information without compromising individual rights to privacy.

- The eligibility criteria should be clarified.

- Recruitment and training of outreach workers should be done by someone skilled in community organization and program planning.

- Sites should put less emphasis on regular attendance and more emphasis on warm welcomes, friendly service, and open invitations to return.

FUTURE DIRECTIONS

Where should we be going with future community nutrition programs for older adults? These programs are certainly an important health promotion activity and especially important to the older adult at high risk for nutritional deficiency. The congregate meal programs are an excellent means of providing nutrition as well as services to older adults. Many issues related to these programs have been discussed and need to be resolved in order to better meet the goals of improving the diets of the participants as well as enhancing feelings of self-esteem and self-reliance.

Another issue that relates to both the congregate meal sites and the home-delivered meals is the need for special diets. At present, the only available diets are regular and low calorie. The low-calorie diet can be adapted to a diabetic diet by the older adult participant who may need some assistance with this. However, since so many older adults are on special diets, it may be helpful to have provision for these various diets, especially low sodium, diabetic, and low cholesterol and fat.

These congregate programs should be improved to better meet the needs of greater numbers of at-risk individuals. This means improved outreach, improved transportation to centers and strategic location centers, more health promotion activities (e.g., screening and assessment), and more innovative nutrition education programs which involve and interest the participants.

Nutrition education for older adults could certainly be expanded via the congregate meal programs and other routes. The recently mandated health and nutrition education demonstration projects are a good start. Older adults can and do change, if motivated and convinced that the change is beneficial and desirable. Lasswell and Curry (1979) designed a pilot program in which a pretest and posttest were used to determine older adults' nutritional knowledge before and after an instruction program. There was a significant difference between the pretest and posttest scores. The investigators pointed out that "the elderly are quite capable of learning new information and changing their belief systems to conform with researched facts rather than myth. The pre- and posttests included items which challenged myths commonly believed about nutrition and health."

Nutrition education for older adults can take many forms in order to reach as many of this population as possible. Within the congregate meal sites, nutrition games as well as discussions may be used. Another nutrition education method used by the Montgomery County Nutrition Project (J. Hubbard & L. King, personal communication, June 28, 1985) is to place nutrition information and recipes on paper placemats. These also reach the homebound elderly with the home-delivered meals. Simply written, informative handouts are useful. Large lettering is a must due to changes in the eyesight of the older adult.

Grotkowski and Sims (1978) asked older adults to identify helpful sources of nutrition education. In descending order of frequency, those named were television, physicians, magazine articles, and cookbooks. Polls have shown that television is a major information source for older adults. For example, the Harris poll found that individuals over age 65 spend more time viewing television than they do reading or listening to the radio (Baran, Briley, & Gillham, 1984). This suggests that television may be a primary way of reaching this age group. Unfortunately, much of the information they receive via the media is on advertisements for snack foods. The information is not very useful. In fact, Clancy (1975) studied the food habits of elderly consumers and found that "the percentage of calories represented by snack foods in the 24-hour recall correlated positively with the number of hours of television the subjects watched daily." A case could be made for attempting to intersperse some sound nutritional messages between the many food advertisements. Both short public service announcements and longer educational programs may be appropriate. The latter is especially feasible for public and cable television. Videotapes are another possible format. However, the lower income individuals, who are at the highest risk, are not reached with videotape and cable television.

An example of a nutrition education television program is "Foodene," developed at Pennsylvania State University (Shannon, Thurman, & Schiff, 1979) This was directed to all age groups, not just older adults. It was an hour long show divided into five segments including the nutrients, dietary fat and heart disease, protein, obesity and weight control, and vitamins. "Foodene" was broadcast on public television. Following the program, a free Food Shopper's Guide was offered to anyone requesting it from the television station. Viewer response was one of the largest the station has had to an instructional program, indicating the high level of interest in the topic. The developers of the program found that the lecture-style presentation was well accepted, but recommended that future programs be shortened to no more than 30 minutes in length.

Although this program was not directed primarily to older adults, this type of format and media may be an excellent way of reaching them. Baran, et al. (1984), in a needs assessment of use of television for older adults, found that they preferred a news/documentary format such as that of "60 Minutes," but preferred a length of 30 minutes rather than 60. The investigators point out that

> this population is in need of substantiative nutritional information, but they are not a helpless audience . . . they are television sophisticates with some nutritional knowledge; therefore, a "show and tell" or "talking head" approach to programming for this group is inappropriate. Factual, informational television, programmed in a manner consistent with the expressed preferences of this audience, would seem to be an ideal way of meeting their nutritional information needs.

Besides television, other areas where efforts toward nutrition education should be made include articles in magazines known to be read by older adults, posters and displays in senior citizen centers, clinics, doctors' offices, and even grocery stores. Efforts need to be made to give accurate, useful information and overcome the many myths, fads, and nutrition misinformation that abounds in the community. This is useful for all age groups; as long as we are looking to the future, let's remember that today's young adults are tomorrow's senior citizens! Additionally, in some situations the young adults are the ones planning meals and cooking for their older relatives. Thus, educational efforts really need to be directed to all age groups.

A media that has not yet been mentioned is the computer. This is probably more appropriate to the young and middle adult audience at present and is still a very selective audience. However, in years to come, this may become a very important method of nutrition planning and education. Some computer-assisted instruction programs in nutrition are already available. Programs could be made available to analyze an individual's nutrient intake, calculate his or her needs, and make recommendations for improvement of nutrient intake. The computer could even become a way of communicating with a health care professional via a computer hook-up.

It must be kept in mind that all the nutritional education in the world will not do the individual any good if he or she is unable to get out to the grocery store or to prepare meals. Thus, transportation to grocery stores, which some senior citizen centers provide, is helpful and needs to be more widely available. Also, homemaker services to assist with shopping and food preparation should be available where needed.

Improved ways of assessing the nutritional status of older adults, identifying their nutritional needs, and using appropriate community resources to meet those needs must be established. Various models of comprehensive, coordinated, multidisciplinary systems have been proposed (Ross Health Administration, 1983). One such model was developed at the Geriatrics Institute at Mt. Sinai Medical Center in Milwaukee (Fish, 1983). Recognizing that older adults have many problems, the goal was to develop a central access point where an older adult could receive all needed services (e.g., medical, nursing, psychosocial, economic, transportation). The program includes rehabilitation, day care, home care, and outreach. This type of comprehensive program provides a point at which an older adult can obtain all services, including nutrition services. For an older adult to attempt to decide what his or her needs are and then where to go for services that meet those needs in an uncoordinated system of community programs can be most confusing. A coordinated program such as that in Milwaukee can alleviate this problem. Funding should be directed to create similar programs in other communities. Appropriate nutrition programs and services would then be a part of the overall comprehensive health system.

Because of the increasing numbers of older adults and earlier hospital discharges, more individuals will require nutrition services. The expansion and coordination of existing nutrition programs for older adults, combined with improved outreach and education, are needed to help these older adults meet their nutritional needs.

The goal is to provide services that assist the older adult to meet his or her own nutritional needs to maintain the highest possible level of wellness. Because independence and self-determination are highly valued, services must be designed to meet identified individual needs rather than encourage dependence. Health assessment programs for older adults are essential in determining what those individual needs are. The availability of a comprehensive health care system for older adults, one that is coordinated with all community services, would be an effective means to identify high-risk individuals and enroll them in the appropriate programs.

REFERENCES

ADA takes a proactive stance, testifies on Older Americans Act reauthorization. (1984). *Journal of the American Dietetic Association, 84,* 822-835.

Albanese, A. (1978). Calcium nutriton in the elderly. *Postgraduate Medicine, 63,* 167-171.

Baran, S., Briley, M., Gillham, M., et al. (1984). Utilizing television to bring nutrition information to the elderly. *Journal of Nutrition for the Elderly, 4*(2)15-25.

Bennett, K. (1984, February) Enteral nutrition: Another option in home care. *Rx Home Care,* p. 42.

Betts, N. M., & Vivian, U.M. (1985) Factors related to the dietary adequacy of noninstitutionalized elderly. *Journal of Nutrition for the Elderly, 4*(4), 3-13.

Chumlea, W., Steinbaugh, M., Roche, A., et al. (1985). Nutritional anthropometric assessment in elderly persons 65 to 90 years of age. *Journal of Nutrition for the Elderly, 4*(4), 39-51.

Clancy, K. Preliminary observations on media use and food habits of the elderly. *The Gerontologist* (1975, December), p. 531.

Fish, A. (1983). Resources and services demanded by the elderly: A community-based approach. In *The Maturity Society in the Maturing Health Care System.* Repsort of the Second Ross Health Administration Forum, Amelia Island, Florida, (pp. 51-56).

Folk, C., & Courtney, M. (1982). Home tube feedings: General guidelines and specific patient instructions. *Nutritional Support Services, 2,* 18.

Freedman, M., & Ahronheim, J. (1985). Nutritional needs of the elderly: Debate and recommendations. *Geriatrics, 40,* 45-59.

Fulwood, R., Johnson, C. L., Bryner, J. D., et al. (1982). *Hemotological and Nutritional Biochemistry Reference Data for Persons 6 Months–74 Years of Age: United States, 1976-1980.* Vital and Health Statistics (series 11, no. 232). U.S. Public Service National Center for Health Services, DHHS Publ. no. PHS 83-1682.

Greene, J. (1981). Coordination of older americans act program. *Journal of the American Dietetic Association, 78,* 617-620.

Grotkowski, M., & Sims, L. (1978). Nutritional knowledge, attitudes, and dietary practices of the elderly. *Journal of the American Dietetic Association, 72,* 502.

Hentzler, J., & Henneman, A. (1980). Where Can You Go for Nutritional Assistance for the Elderly? *Journal of Gerontological Nursing, 6,* 551-552.

Hickler, R. B. (1984). Nutrition and the elderly. *Academy of Family Practice, 29,* 137-145.

Holdsworth, M. D., & Davies, L. (1982). Nutrition education for the elderly. *Human Nutrition, 36,* 22-27.

Kennedy, Senator E. M. (1983). Going hungry in America. *Report to the Committee on Labor and Human Resources,* U.S. Senate.

Lasswell, A., & Curry, K. (1979). Curriculum development of instructing the elderly in nutrition. *Journal of Nutritional Education, 11,* 14.

Mobile Meals, Inc. (1982-1983). *Annual Report.* Akron, Ohio.

Munro, H., and Young, V. (1978). Protein metabolism in the elderly. *Postgraduate Medicine, 63,* 143-152.

National Academy of Sciences. (1980). *Recommended Dietary Allowances* (9th ed.). Washington, DC.

Pear, Robert. (1985, September 23). Lower nutrient levels proposed in draft report on American diet. *New York Times.*

Ross Health Administration, Report of the Second Forum. (1983). *The Maturing Society in the Maturing Health Care System,* Amelia Island, Florida.

Schneider, R. (1979). Barriers to effective outreach in Title VII nutrition programs. *The Gerontologist, 19,* 163-168.

Shannon, B., Thurman, G., & Schiff, W. (1979). Foodene: A pilot TV show on nutrition issues. *Journal of Nutrition Education, 11,* 15-18.

U.S. Department of Health, Education, and Welfare. (1977). *Dietary Intake Finding, United States, 1971-1974.* (Publication No. HRA 77I-1647). National Center for Health Statistics.

U.S. Department of Health, Education, and Welfare. (1972). *Center for Disease Control: Ten-State Nutrition Survey, 1968-1970: V. Dietary.* (Publication No. HSM 72-8133). Atlanta, Georgia.

U.S. Department of Health and Human Services. (1984). *Older Americans Act of 1965,* as amended, P.L. 98-459.

U.S. Department of Health and Human Services. (1984). *Older Americans Act of 1965,* as amended, Title III, Part A, Section 307 (p. 27).

Wateska, L., Sattler, L., & Steigler, E. (1980). Cost of a home parenteral nutrition program. *Journal of the American Medical Association, 244,* 2303-2304.

STUDY QUESTIONS

1. What factors, either in the individual or in the community, may contribute to the older adult's nutritional status?

2. What purposes do the Title III-C nutrition sites serve? Consider some ways that older adults in these centers could benefit from nursing involvement.

3. What are some ways in which your community has provided for the nutritional care of homebound older adults. What are some alternative ways the community could provide that nutritional care?

4. How might your community plan and implement nutrition education programs for older adults in the community?

5. What types of research questions need to be answered in order to better identify the nutritional needs of older adults and also to provide data that may be influential in obtaining adequate funding for coordinated, comprehensive nutrition programs?

7 PROFESSIONAL AND PUBLIC EDUCATION INITIATIVES: ADDRESSING HEALTH AND RELATED NEEDS OF ELDERLY PERSONS

Sister Rose Therese Bahr, PhD, FAAN

HEALTH AND RELATED NEEDS OF ELDERLY PERSONS

The population of Americans who are 65 years of age and over is growing at a phenomenal rate. America is becoming a nation with the largest population of older persons in the world. In 1983 the median age of the population reached 30.9 years, the oldest ever, and is expected to exceed 36 years by the year 2000. A recent report ("Snapshot," 1985) cited there were more Americans over the age of 65 than there were teenagers. This change is rapidly altering the American health care industry.

To appreciate the particulars of this new statistical orientation, an overview of the current population is provided here from an information paper by the U.S. Senate Special Committee on Aging titled *America in Transition: An Aging Society, 1984-85 edition.* This publication reflects the demographic distribution, economic status, health status, and health services utilization of the current population of older adults.

Geographic Distribution

- Over one-half of elderly persons live in just eight states: California, New York, Florida, Pennsylvania, Texas, Illinois, Ohio, and Michigan.

- In 1980, for the first time, more elderly persons lived in the suburbs than in central cities.

- On the average, older persons change residences half as often as younger persons.

- Older persons who move out of state tend to move to the Sunbelt. The number of Americans moving to the Sunbelt who are age 60 or older has nearly doubled since 1950.

- A new trend called *countermigration* has emerged in which some persons 60 years of age or older who migrated to the Sunbelt in their early retirement years return to their home states or to the homes of family or friends.

Economic Status

- Older persons have substantially less cash income than those under 65 years of age. In 1983, the median income of a family head 65 years or older was less than two-thirds the median income of a family head age 25–64 years.

- Elderly persons are more likely than other adults to be poor. In 1983, 14.1 percent of persons age 65 years and older had incomes below the poverty level, compared to 12.1 percent of those age 18–64 years and 15.4 percent of all persons under age 65.

- The old old (85 years of age and older) have significantly lower money incomes than the young old (65–74 years of age). In 1983 the median cash income of couples aged 85 and over ($11,988) was less than three-quarters the median cash income of couples aged 65–74 ($17,798).

- In 1983, the median income of elderly women was slightly more than half the median income of elderly men—$5,599 versus $9,766. Nearly three-quarters of the elderly poor population are women.

- Non-white elderly individuals have substantially lower money incomes than their white counterparts. For instance, among those aged 65–69, white males had a median income of $12,180 compared to a median of $7,097 for black men, and $6,551 for hispanic men.

- The elderly rely heavily on Social Security benefits and asset income. In 1982, 39 percent of all income received by aged household units came from Social Security and 25 percent came from assets income.

- In recent decades Social Security and assets have grown as a source of income for the elderly, while earnings have become less important. Between 1968 and 1983, the share of income for elderly families provided by Social Security grew from 23.9 to 43.3 percent of income and the share provided by asset income from 14.6 to 20.9 percent. At the same time, the share contributed by earnings fell from 48.2 to 28 percent.

Health Status and Health Services Utilization

- Contrary to stereotype, most older persons view their health positively. Even if they have a chronic illness, four out of five elderly describe their health as good or excellent compared to others their own age.

- One out of five elderly have at least a mild degree of disability.

- Over one-half of the oldest old have no physical disability, but the chance of becoming disabled increases with age.

- Cross-sectional data has shown that the likelihood of having a chronic illness increases with age. More than four out of five persons 65 years of age and over have at least one chronic condition and multiple conditions are commonplace.

- Many psychiatric problems are not as common for older persons as for younger persons. However, the primary health problem of older age is cognitive impairment, which can be related to a number of sources, including Alzheimer's disease. A recent study has shown that 14 percent of the elderly have at least a mild form of cognitive impairment.

- Three out of four elderly persons die from heart disease, cancer or stroke. Though heart disease is declining, it remains the major cause of death today.

- Death rates, a statistical measure of the frequency of death in the population, reached an all-time low in 1983.

- "Informal supports," the help of friends, spouses, and other relatives, provide valuable assistance to elderly persons in the community. For instance, in 1982, relatives provided approximately 80 percent of all community care to disabled elderly men.

- Only about 5 percent of the elderly live in nursing homes at any given time. In 1985, an estimated 11.5 million elderly persons will reside in nursing homes.

- The elderly are the heaviest users of health services. They account for 19 percent of all hospital discharges and one-third of the country's personal health care expenditures, even though they constitute only 11 percent of the population. Health care utilization is also greatest in the last year of life and among the old old.

- Out-of-pocket health expenses for the elderly are now the same as they were prior to the enactment of Medicare and Medicaid. Today, the average out of the pocket expense is $1,058 annually.

- Per capita spending for health care for the elderly was $4,202 in 1984.

The health care needs of the aging adult as demonstrated in this overview suggest an aging individual who wishes to be independent and accountable, to receive the same dignity and respect accorded to any other individual, and to be recognized as one who is making a contribution to society. From a health perspective, the older person's positive attitude toward life and his healthy state through implementation and continuation of health care practices is wholesome, satisfying, and life giving.

However, physical and cognitive disabilities have a tendency to increase as the person ages. The aged individual who may suffer from the deteriorating condition of Alzheimer's disease is particularly vulnerable. Heart disease, cancer, and stroke are the most debilitating for the elderly individual. Friends, spouses, relatives, and neighbors provide the major portion of informal support to maintain the elderly person in the home and functioning at an optimal level.

Two important observations in this report are that (1) the majority of elderly persons who live in the community attempt to continue a life-style that has allowed them to reach an advanced age, and (2) it is the "frail" elderly group that is the fastest growing segment of the population and requires the greatest amount of health care from an institution (U.S. Special Committee, 1985).

The health needs of the older person include the totality of personal needs or the universal self-care needs as delineated in Orem's self-care theory. These universal needs for total health include:

- maintenance of sufficient intake of air, water, food.

- proper maintenance of elimination processes.

- maintenance of balance between activity and rest, solitude and social interaction.

- elimination of any barriers that may interfere with human functioning and well-being.

- activation of human functioning and development within social groups in achievement of one's human potential to live life normally* (Orem, 1980).

Related needs of the elderly person are psychosocial-spiritual and include:

- The need to be seen as an individual, not a stereotypic myth.

- The need to be involved in planned activities with maintenance of decision-making powers.

- The need to be affirmed in one's individuality and to receive acceptance of whatever lifestyle is chosen.

- The need to be creative in the expression of behaviors according to one's personality and social values.

- The need to be perceived as a spiritual human being who needs to be loved, touched, and given positive regard for self.

Health and related needs that are fulfilled allow for a fully functioning life with full decision-making powers. This independent and autonomous life is

---

* *Nursing, Concepts of Practice,* 2nd ed. (p. 42) by D. Orem, 1980, St. Louis: McGraw-Hill. Copyright 1980 by McGraw-Hill. Reproduced by permission.

the goal of every aging person, and it should guide health professionals as they engage in health-related activities with the older adult. Unfortunately, lack of knowledge regarding the aging processes, health promotion, and maintenance of older adults is so prevalent that it hinders the fulfillment of their health needs.

CURRENT STATUS OF PROFESSIONAL AND PUBLIC EDUCATION

Public Education

Public education initiatives, which exceed professional initiatives, are being implemented through a variety of models. During the past ten years, lobbying efforts by the American Association of Retired Persons (AARP), the Grey Panthers, church groups, and other organizations concerned about the elderly population in America, have resulted in the implementation of many formal and informal models of public education through various media. These programs present information on a variety of issues and topics pertinent to the older population and the general public. The content is derived from current research projects which generate scientific findings about various diseases, preventive health measures, and promotion of a more positive attitude toward the aging process and the older person in society.

Television and Radio Programs. Models of public education have used various techniques and methodologies within the community to educate the consumer about health and related needs of older adults. Programs such as the daily CNN health news; "Over Easy", with Ted Downs; radio and television talk shows with older artists, musicians, and actors who are 60 years of age and over; and movies such as *On Golden Pond* that depict life in the later years present just a few of the many opportunities to promote public education for and about aging.

Printed Materials. Models of public education are also present in society in printed literature distributed by many organizations. One of the main contributors of such material is AARP. Booklets published in 1985 by this Washington, D.C.,-based organization include *Truth About Aging: Guidelines for Accurate Communication; A Consumer Education Bibliography for Older*

Americans; Organizing Educational Seminars: A How-to Guide and the *Educational and Service Programs* booklet that describes the broad range of services available to the older American within the community. The *Community Programs Idea Book: A Volunteer's Guide* includes information on consumer rights, widowed persons services, citizen representation, financial planning, and health services available to older adults. This organization distributes free pamphlets on all aspects of health and related needs. The pamphlets contain many suggestions on health care and available services.

Recently the AARP endorsed four major initiatives to be implemented over the next five years that would expand options and enhance the quality of life for the older individuals in America. These initiatives include:

1. *Healthy U.S.* Healthy U.S. was started to address the increasing problem facing the nation's entire health care system. Its goals are to (1) reduce the rate of cost escalation in all kinds of health care, (2) preserve and strengthen the Medicare and Medicaid program, (3) encourage the development of alternative health delivery systems, (4) encourage Americans of all ages to develop more healthful life-styles, and (5) provide information about health care costs and options to consumers.

2. *Minority Affairs Initiative.* The goal of the Minority Affairs Initiative is to create greater awareness of the special needs and concerns of, and conditions faced by older minority persons. It addresses the underlying causes of those conditions through issues-oriented advocacy and by developing new approaches to meet the needs of racial and ethnic minorities. It also draws attention to the positive contributions of minority persons to American life.

3. *Older Women's Advocacy Initiative.* The Older Women's Advocacy Initiative endeavors to strengthen and enlarge the leadership roles held by women. It addresses the special health, financial, and social needs that midlife and older women must fulfill to realize their full potential, and focuses attention on the contributions women are making to society.

4. *Older Workers Advocacy Initiative.* The Older Workers Advocacy Initiative addresses the issues surrounding an aging workforce and seeks to expand work options available to older persons. Part of this initiative is securing preretirement planning programs that employers and organizations can sponsor for employees.

Government Programs. The National Health Promotion initiative recently implemented by the United States Administration on Aging and the United States Public Health Service encourages states and local communities to develop health promotion activities for older persons. The initiative is designed to (1) enhance the quality of life for older Americans through the improvement of their health status and preservation of their independence, (2) focus attention on health promotion and disease prevention, especially in the areas of injury control, proper drug use, better nutrition, and improved physical fitness, and (3) curtail health costs caused by preventable conditions. A publication entitled *A Healthy Old Age: A Sourcebook for Health Promotion for Older Adults* describes the process for organizing and conducting health promotion activities at the community level (U.S. Administration on Aging and Public Health Service, 1984).

College Programs. Another model of public education is the college degree-granting program in community colleges. This initiative is designed to help the older adult to learn about and meet his or her needs. An example of such a program, which is properly titled "60-Plus," was initiated in 1980 in a four-year college in Kansas. Older adults may enroll part-time at reduced tuition in courses leading to a degree. Recently, a 73-year-old retired businessman obtained a BS in psychology "to better understand myself and my world." He plans to use this knowledge in a position counseling older adults in his church.

Workshops and Conferences. Models of public education are in effect in workshops, teleconferences, circuit courses, institutes, seminars, and conferences. These models are free to the public, and educate them on health and related needs of the older person. Slowly, society's attitude toward the older adult is becoming one of tolerance and limited acceptance. Much work remains for the public education service organizations. They must continue thier attempts to reduce the prejudices and biases against an individual purely because he or she has lived a longer life. A small breakthrough has occured in the upgrading of the health status of older adults through public education.

Professional Education

In 1965 at the historical moment created by the American Nurses' Association (ANA) for promotion of the educational preparation of the nurse into the mainstream of higher education, another momentous idea was enacted. That idea was the creation of the Division of Geriatric Nursing and is now known as the Council on Gerontological Nursing. For the first time, the ANA House of Delegates brought visibility to the aging population who were in need of health care in various settings. This newly created organizational unit immediately promoted the role of the gerontological/geriatric nurse through development of a philosophy of gerontological nursing, identification of the scope of this new specialty, and projection of the standards of its practice.

Initiatives underway as goals of the Council of Gerontological Nursing reported in the Council's Newsletter, *Oasis* (1984) include:

1. Development of a comprehensive data base to support the council's positions to help in the planning of program activities (e.g.,

gerontological nurse specialist certification program).
2. Revision of the scope and standards of gerontological nursing practice.
3. Promotion of high standards of gerontological nursing practice.
4. Advancement of gerontological nursing to a significant specialty in the field of aging.

This Council, however honorable and noble its intentions, was unable to accomplish a greatly increased understanding and acceptance by nurses of gerontological/geriatric nursing as an enriching and rewarding career alternative. It continues to be as much of a struggle today as it was in 1965 even though the need has increased because the population of older adults has almost doubled in size.

Graduate Nursing Programs.   In the 1970s, monies from the Division of Nursing assisted in establishing specialty tracks in gerontological nursing in university setting. However, there were few teachers who were qualified and had credentials. Most of these gerontological nursing tracks were administered and taught by faculty who prepared themselves through short-term continuing education programs, institutes, or summer courses for credit. Few students took advantage of the master's degree programs in gerontological nursing because they were reluctant to choose this less-recognized professional track. Some universities received the monies, implemented a program, but failed to make a full commitment to the preparation of gerontological nurse specialists or geriatric nurse practitioners. Consequently, after the grant monies terminated, a number of the programs also terminated because of a lack of faculty and student interest. Some remaining programs offer a few gerontological nursing courses but not a full-fledged gerontological nursing program. Others provide a full concentration that prepares students for the certification examination under the auspices of the ANA.

The nurse practitioner programs have expanded the most since 1970. In 1970 there were approximately 36 nurse practitioner programs with 250 students compared to 193 programs with almost 2,269 students in 1981 (Sultz, 1983). The number of nurse practitioner programs specifically training geriatric nurses has increased from approximately 15 programs in 1980 to 35 programs in 1985. However, there are only 218 geriatric nurse practitioners certified by the ANA, compared to the 6,215 adult and family nurse practitioners (ANA, 1984). Thus, geriatric nursing continues to have problems recruiting students because of the poor image, prestige, and pay involved in such a career choice.

According to Capezuti (1985) in a survey conducted of nine geriatric nurse practitioner programs in the Northeast only one program required clinical experience in long-term home health care agency for an entire semester. In the remaining eight programs only some students received home care experiences, yet that setting encompasses the majority of the elderly today. Since most older people do not wish to be institutionalized, the geriatric nurse practitioner and gerontological nurse specialist must be aware of all resources that help the older person to live a high quality of life in the community.

Undergraduate Nursing Programs. Undergraduate programs in nursing also have a major problem in addressing the health needs of the older adult. Little or no content is being included in the curricula for nursing student regarding the health and related needs of the aging in the community or institution. Although the National League for Nursing, Council of Baccalaureate and Higher Degree Programs Criterion 24 for accreditation delineates the need for this content, educators and faculty have been slow to respond to this additional requirement in a highly visible way. Most educators in baccalaureate nursing programs are indicating that the course content on aging is integrated within the curricular offerings of the program. Yet, upon close examination, little content is found. Some schools may include a one hour lecture on the aging person in the community; others may use the nursing home for a nursing arts laboratory where students practice the nursing skills on elderly bed-confined individuals. But an organized approach to content on the aging process and specific developmental and health needs of the elderly is not uniformly included in all programs.

Faculty, with lack of commitment to care of the aging person, are most reluctant to place students in settings where the majority of recipients of care are elderly. Deans of baccalaureate, master's and doctoral degree programs in nursing have not made a total commitment to the need for establishment of departments of gerontological/geriatric nursing within colleges of nursing, even though statistics show that the United States is a graying nation and that nursing has a mandate from society to minister to its health needs. Students returning to school are older than they were ten years ago. But the fact remains, little heed is being given to the needs of the older adult within baccalaureate nursing programs.

FUTURE INITIATIVES: PROFESSIONAL AND PUBLIC EDUCATION

Initiatives in Education and Service

What, then, are some of the initiatives and models of education needed in the future to meet the needs of elderly adults? Education follows the trends in the service area. If this is true, then the initiatives for professional and public education must examine the service models being tested and implemented in the community in an attempt to meet the needs of the elderly.

A new initiative that has implications for professional education and curriculum offerings is the model of nurse practitioner utilization in home care currently being marketed by Health Options in the northeast. Contracting with individual and group-practice physicians as well as health maintenance organizations to make home visits to patients who are homebound and have been recently discharged from the hospital, or to acutely ill people who are at home but do not require hospitalization, is being tested as a way to deliver better nursing care to the older adults in the community. In addition to regular home visits, services are offered during the evening, night, and weekend periods, when most agencies are not available to the patients. Another option being explored is for the geriatric nurse practitioners to contract with family members who live long distances from older relatives and who wish to receive reports from health professionals regarding the older persons' health status.

One of the major groups to face an onslaught of aging individuals on a nationwide scale into their health care system is the Veterans Administration. This organization has determined that the peak of its aging population will occur in the year 2000. There is much discussion among multidisciplinary groups in this agency on determining the strategies needed to meet the critical needs in the future. According to Ferguson some of the initiatives suggested include:

1. Formulate a master plan for long-term care of aging individuals within the institution and the community-based care facilities within the next three to five years so that it is clear who is in charge of the care of aging persons at what point in the health care delivery system.

2. Increase the number of gerontological nursing programs which prepare clinical nurse specialists and nurse practitioners for community, nursing home, and hospital-based and home care so that a continuum of care is in place for the care of the aging person in whatever setting and at whatever level of care is necessary.

3. Promote the establishment of departments of gerontological/geriatric nursing in all schools of nursing to give visibility to this area of nursing as a specialty. This, in turn, would act as a recruitment device for potential nurses seeking a career track in nursing or a possible retrenchment of nurses seeking a second career in nursing.

4. Attach more prestige to the area of gerontological nursing by sophisticated public relations programs about the quality of care given by nurse gerontologist. A greatly publicized awards system would be one strategy.

5. Promote collegial relationships and support groups among qualified professional nurses by encouraging health care agencies and institutions to employ a group of nurses so that these professionals

continue their educational enrichment while in service to others.

Cynthia Cieplik, (personal communication, August 27, 1985) council services staff specialist of the American Nurses' Association, notes that initiatives being pursued by the Council of Gerontological Nursing within the next five years bear heavily on the professional educational component. Elected leaders who are nurse gerontologists in the council are examining the vast differences among educators regarding their definitions of gerontological nursing, the scope of their practice, their competency requirements and their standards of practice in gerontological nursing. Initiatives projected for the future include:

1. Consensus-building events conducted in a variety of configurations so that meetings organized on a local or regional basis could be brought to a national meeting. Current data on charcteristics of gerontological nursing practice among diverse settings and populations are needed to enhance the documents used in a wide distribution for interpreting gerontological nursing in multidisciplinary groups.

    This initiative could serve to develop strategies that foster adequate numbers of appropriately prepared nurse practitioners in the field of gerontological nursing and to link education preparation to the essential elements of needed gerontological services in both institutional and community-based settings (C. Cieplik, personal communication, 1985).

2. Establishing additional doctoral programs with focus on research in the areas of gerontological nursing.

3. Conducting more research to demonstrate models of health care more conducive to the holistic health orientation for maintenance of a high quality of life for the aging individual.

4. Promoting inclusion of a special course in gerontological nursing in all baccalaureate nursing curricula.

5. Preparing specialists who can take leadership in the provision of multiple health care services for the elderly population.

6. Emphasizing interdisciplinary health care services and working with volunteers and others to assure the spread of such services.

7. Promoting continuing education in gerontological nursing through teleconferences, circuit courses, workshops, and conferences.

8. Exploring models of service and education to address the needs

of the elderly population in the community (C. Cieplik, personal communication, 1985).

The entire range of human services is needed to meet the demands for care of chronically ill aged persons. Services needed range from medical care, nursing care, psychiatric and mental health care, hospitalization, nursing home care, home health care, hospice care, day care, personal care, homemaking, environmental maintenance, meals, transportation, dental care, and family assistance including counseling and respite care. The goal of these services is to allow the aging person to function optimally from a health perspective (ANA, 1983).

Models of Professional and Public Education

Models of practice for professional and public education for the future were projected by the task force cited above. The five models included:

Model 1. Primary providers of service would include a physician, a nurse, and home service workers who would provide medical services, skilled home nursing services, home health aide services, and social services. The recipients of this care would be frail aged persons including those with loss of mental function; recently discharged persons requiring convalescent care and readaptation to community living; persons in temporarily unstable situations such as grief, retirement, relocation, sensory loss, and terminal illness or dying. This model would supplement the type of traditional care modalities presently in organizations such as the Visiting Nurse Association (VNA) and the other organized health care delivery systems.

Model 2. The social health maintenance organization is designed to address problems of (1) unnecessary reliance on institutional and medical care for problems which require other types of interventions; (2) the separation between the medical and social care of the elderly, and (3) the open-ended fee-for-service nature of reimbursement. The objective of the social health maintenance organization is to extend the concepts of prevention, early detection, and early treatment to a frail, chronically ill, at-risk elderly population.

Model 3. The purpose of the Block Nurse Program for the Aged is to provide local, community-based nursing services to older residents that enable them to remain in their home for as long as possible. Services are provided by nurses who reside in the community and can be easily reached by residents on a 24-hour basis. The focus of services on health maintenance and promotion is intended to maintain the older individual in his home and avoid unnecessary or premature institutionalization.

Model 4. In this model the nurse would be the coordinator of care in the nursing home. This would establish comprehensive and planned health maintenance and health promotion activities. Communication with the individual's physician would coordinate needed medical care and support early intervention to prevent unnecessary hospitalization and to obtain acute care/hospital services when they are needed.

Model 5. Primary care ambulatory clinics could more efficiently coordinate the multiple care requirements of this population and facilitate a more organized access to other supportive services. This model could accommodate both cooperative physician-nurse practice and nurse-administered clinics. Appropriate mechanisms for interfacing with physicians in specialty practice and other providers would need to be determined and facilitated throughout the larger system.

Each of the community-based practice models demands educational programs to prepare health professionals for these care modalities to meet the health and related needs of the elderly population. Meeting these needs will allow the older adult to maintain a healthy, self-reliant, self-determined lifestyle satisfying to each of them on all dimensions, (i.e., physical, social, psychological and spiritual). Much needs to be accomplished to persuade various constituencies to initiate a series of programs in a well-planned and organized approach to overcoming ageism in the long-term care industry, the community, and the institution. Through such activities the master plan of care for the older adult could become a reality in the foreseeable future. Agencies and agents who should be encouraged to become partners with nurses in the overcoming of ageism include:

1. *Congress.* Congress should provide monies for the establishment of gerontological nursing departments, curriculum development, student recruitment and stipends, building the body of knowledge through research, evaluation to continually identify further components of knowledge and skills needed by practitioners in the field of aging.

2. *School officials, deans of nursing programs, and faculties.* They should accept the field of gerontological nursing as a specialty and increase its visibility in curricular offerings.

3. *The public.* They should maintain a reality-based approach to the academic focus in the field of gerontological nursing.

Some positive efforts in the public and professional arenas of education have begun to effect better care for aging individuals in the United States. However, much needs to be done to ensure that all aging persons in whatever setting may obtain the needed services and care by professionals who are qualified by education to assume the responsibility for this awesome task. Both society and the nursing and medical professions cannot wait. Each day brings more and more aging persons into the fragmented system of care that is presently in place. Efforts on the behalf of aging persons cannot slacken now.

REFERENCES

American Nurses' Association. (1983). *AMA/ANA Task Force to Address the Improvement of Health Care of the Aged Chronically Ill.*

American Nurses' Association Council of Gerontological Nursing. (1984). *Oasis,* p. 3.

American Nurses' Association/Kansas. (1984). *American Nurses' Association 1984 certification catalog.* Kansas City, MO: Kansas Association.

Capezuti, E. (1985). Geriatric nurse practitioners: Their education, experience and future in home health care. *Pride Institute Journal of Long Term Home Health Care 4,* 9-14.

Ferguson. (1985). *The Olivian* Washington, DC: The Catholic University of America School of Nursing, p. 2.

Kane, R. (1981). *Geriatrics in the United States manpower projections and training considerations. MA: Lexington Books.*

Mountain State Health Corporation. (1985). *Gerontological nurse practitioner educational directory.* Boise, ID: Mountain State Health Corporation.

Orem, D. (1980). *Nursing: Concepts of practice* (2nd ed.). St. Louis: McGraw-Hill.

Snapshot of a changing america. (1985, September 2). *Newsweek,* p. 16.

Sultz, H. (1983). *Study of nurse practitioners programs, students, graduates and employers of nurse practitioners.* Springfield, VA: Services.

The Challenge. (1985). Wichita, KS: Kansas Newman College Press.

United States Administration on Aging and USPHS. (1984). *A healthy old age: A sourcebook for health promotion for older Americans.* Washington, DC: U.S. Government Printing Office.

United States Senate Special Committee on Aging. (1985). *America in transition: An aging society, 1984-85 edition.* Washington, DC: U.S. Government Printing Office, 1-4.

STUDY QUESTIONS

1. What are the major geographic distributions of elderly persons in American society today and what impact has this phenomenon had on health care for the elderly?

2. What are the major health and related needs of aging persons in our nation?

3. What are the universal self-care needs enumerated by Orem's theory?

4. What is the present status of public education on aging and the aged population regarding health and related needs?

5. What are the major problems in professional education today regarding preparation of health professionals to meet the needs of older adults?

6. How can some of the projected models for health delivery for older persons improve their health needs?

7. Who should become partners to bring about change in the public and professional educational arena and enhance health care needs of the older adult?

RECOMMENDATIONS

Only 5 to 20 percent of elderly people are ever admitted into long-term care at any one time. The percentage increases and the need intensifies as the accumulation of chronic illnesses interferes with the elderly individual's functional independence. The 80 to 95 percent of elderly persons who remain in the community have varying levels of need to maintain their level of independence. While the majority of necessary services are provided by family, friends, or other informal caretakers, a large number of formal caregivers and managers will be needed to meet the future needs. It is to this group that these suggestions are directed.

Nursing professionals must prepare themselves and the staff for whom they are responsible, to meet the challenges and opportunities of working with the increasing numbers of elderly persons. Programs in basic and continuing education must provide students with the knowledge and skills to plan, organize, and deliver care to individuals whose needs are within the continuum of community-based and institutional services.

NURSING SERVICE

There is a need for (1) development of a *model for continuity of care* that includes identification of patterns of inpatient referrals, assessment of client and environment with linkage to appropriate resources, establishment of a profile of users of day care and home care to determine collaboration between both providers, and the combination of day care and home care, (2) identification of the appropriate "case manager" on the continuum of care, (3) an increase in staff awareness of the need for out-of-institution services and organizations for the aging population, (4) continuing education of current registered nurses and other nursing personnel in long-term care of the aging,

79

and (5) increased cooperation between the provider industry and the education system to provide scholarships in gerontological nursing, demonstration practice settings, and summer internships for nursing students.

NURSING EDUCATION

1.   A positive image of nursing the aging population must be created.

2.   Measures must be instituted to increase the visibility of gerontological nursing as a major content area in the curriculum at all levels of nursing.

3.   A meeting should be planned with the deans of nursing programs to discuss

   •   The gerontological nursing curriculum content.

   •   The relationship of curriculum content to the accreditation criteria.

   •   The current lack of reference to gerontological nursing on the state board examinations for registered nursing.

   •   The need for emphasis on the cultural dimensions of the elderly population—especially Asian and Hispanic minorities.

   •   The need to expand student experiences in long-term care.

4.   Resources (grants, etc.) available for study and projects in gerontological nursing need to be identified, publicized, and marketed.

5.   Educators need to identify potential linkages with the industry.

PUBLIC EDUCATION

1.   There is a need to broaden the consumers' and the caregivers' knowledge of the availability of alternative services and the changing roles of all family members as the aging process occurs.

2.   Nurses should be available to participate in nationwide education regarding care of the aging and long-term care.

RESEARCH

There is need to

1. Determine the value of exchange between acute care staff and long-term care staff; whether there will be a raise in consciousness regarding long-term care; whether there will be an increase in excellence of care.

2. Identify and measure value-related behaviors in nursing regarding long-term care: patients, organizational approaches, natural versus pathological aging.

3. Determine how to raise the consciousness of deans and faculty to include gerontological content in basic curriculum.

4. Study costing out long-term care nursing settings and interventions.

5. Gain better knowledge of nutritional needs of the elderly population and of how these needs are being met in food growth, accessing, processing, and distribution.

6. Study reasons for the drop-off in congregate meal settings.

7. Determine the health and service needs of the affluent elderly population.

8. Determine the characteristics of day care recipients.

COLLABORATION

1. The NLN Long-Term Care Committee should convey to the American Association of Retired Persons, Gray Panthers, Older Women's League, and so forth its need for help and collaboration, in specific areas of need such as supporting NLN and giving direction in nursing issues affecting older Americans.

2. The NLN Long-Term Care Committee should inform the Tri-Council and the International Council on Nursing Statistics of the need for a data base and collection of data regarding long-term care nursing.

3. Nurses must collaborate with other groups that affect the quality of living for the elderly. These groups include community planners, architects, local safety service groups, county and state planning groups, and financial community planners.

DISCUSSION

The following issues need to be explored in order to effect public policy decisions:

- Reimbursement of nurses.

- Reimbursement issues in institutions that affect levels of care, who can receive care, and so forth.

- Individual rights and responsibilities.

- Shift toward wellness/prevention care.

- Marketing of nursing.

- Physical and psychological abuse of elderly persons.

- Community nursing centers.

- Loss of block grants for the care of elderly persons.

- 1984 Amendment to the Older Persons Act.

- 202 Section 8 Housing—Where are the funds?